Acts of abuse

NORTH CAROLINA
STATE BOARD OF COMMUNITY COLLEGES
LIBRARIES
NASH COMMUNITY COLLEGE

D0645753

Sexual crime is very much in the news, and public fear of rape and sexual abuse has almost become a panic. Practitioners, politicians and the media constantly debate its causes and the best methods of dealing with those sex offenders who are caught and convicted. Yet this debate is often fuelled by ignorance and prejudice, with little understanding of the reality of sexual crime.

Acts of Abuse explores the response of the criminal justice system to the explosion of interest in sexual crime. It examines the existing research about the causes of rape and child abuse, the number of offences being committed, and the policy of the courts. It then analyses the responses of the probation service and the prison system to the increased number of offenders with whom they are being required to deal.

Written by a prominent critic of the British penal system, *Acts of Abuse* is the first comprehensive survey of the phenomenon of sexual crime in the British penal context. It will appeal to students and all professionals working in crime and justice.

Previously an academic and probation officer, **Adam Sampson** is Deputy Director of the Prison Reform Trust.

Related titles available from Routledge:

Crime, Criminal Justice and the Probation Service
Robert Harris

Racism and Anti-Racism in Probation
David Denney

Prisons after Woolf
Reform through riot
Edited by Elaine Player and Michael Jenkins

Women, Policing and Male Violence
International perspectives
Edited by Jalna Hanmer, Jill Radford and Elizabeth A. Stanko

Acts of abuse

Sex offenders and the criminal justice system

Adam Sampson

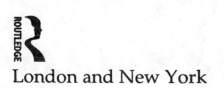

London and New York

First published 1994
by Routledge
11 New Fetter Lane, London EC4P 4EE

Simultaneously published in the USA and Canada
by Routledge
29 West 35th Street, New York, NY 10001

© 1994 Adam Sampson

Typeset in Palatino by LaserScript, Mitcham, Surrey
Printed and bound in Great Britain by
Biddles Ltd, Guildford and King's Lynn

All rights reserved. No part of this book may be reprinted or
reproduced or utilized in any form or by any electronic,
mechanical, or other means, now known or hereafter
invented, including photocopying and recording, or in any
information storage or retrieval system, without permission in
writing from the publishers.

British Library Cataloguing in Publication Data
A catalogue record for this book is available from the British Library.

Library of Congress Cataloging in Publication Data
Sampson, Adam, 1960–
  Acts of abuse: sex offenders and the criminal justice system/
  Adam Sampson.
  p. cm.
  Includes bibliographical references and index.
  1. Sex offenders – Great Britain. 2. Criminal justice,
  Administration of – Great Britain. I. Title.
  HQ72.G7S36   1994
  364.1'53'092241 – dc20   93-17215
                                                            CIP

ISBN 0–415–07372–3 (hbk)
ISBN 0–415–07373–1 (pbk)

For My Father

Erratum

The publishers and author accept that paragraph 3 of page 81 of this publication is incorrect and apologize for any embarrassment caused to any member or officer of Northumbria Probation Service. In particular, Northumbria Probation Service does not wilfully seek to avoid formal (or any other) co-operation. In July 1990, the Northumbria Probation Service appointed a Senior Probation Officer to develop the work of the Service with sex offenders and to examine the possibility of inter-agency and inter-disciplinary co-operation. The Service funded the appointment of two Probation Officers to develop the work within the Service and a steering group of representatives from a variety of agencies and disciplines came together in November 1990. Funding was obtained from three charities. The steering group became the 'Derwent Initiative' whose aim is to promote an inter-agency response to sexual offending and a Director was appointed in August 1992, his appointment being funded by the three charities.

Contents

Acknowledgements

It is *de rigueur* at the start of books like this to offer thanks to the various individuals without whose help . . . etc., etc. In this case, such thanks are more than mere politeness. Much of the information on which this book is based was only made available through the kindness of others. Many individuals listened to my half-formed thoughts on the subject of sexual crime – some even appeared interested – and were prepared to offer advice or point me in the direction of vital source material. Prison and probation staff were willing to discuss their ideas and problems. Offenders were prepared to detail their offences to an inquisitive stranger. And, perhaps most important, survivors of sexual crime consented to revisit their sufferings for my benefit. To all these, my thanks.

However, my thanks are particularly owing to my colleagues at the Prison Reform Trust, and to the two individuals, Stephen Shaw of PRT and Ruth Mann of HMP Wandsworth, who waded through earlier drafts of the text. Needless to say, the mistakes and misunderstandings which remain are mine, and mine alone.

Introduction

We are living in an age when sexual crime dominates the headlines. Scarcely a week goes by without the national newspapers carrying some story of rape, child abuse, or sexual misdemeanour: the allegations of mass rape in the former Yugoslavia; the rape trials of William Kennedy Smith and Mike Tyson in the USA; the continuing saga of Operation Orchid, the massive police investigation of allegations of the murder of tens of boys by a sadistic paedophile ring; the career-ending arrests of the Director of Public Prosecutions and a Conservative MP after allegations of sexual solicitation; the controversy about the existence or otherwise of satanic child abuse; and the events of Rochdale, Cleveland and the Orkneys.

This catalogue of crime has inevitably had its impact upon the public. Public concern about sexual crime has become panic. Women increasingly see themselves at risk of sexual assault, and rape now heads the list of crimes which the public characterizes as serious.[1] Those who perpetrate such crimes are hated and despised more than almost any other offender. Built up into modern folk-devils by the popular press, their treatment at the hands of many people working in the criminal justice system reflects their sub-human status in the popular mind. In the words of a prison officer opening the gate to a sex offenders unit in Wormwood Scrubs: 'Here be monsters'.[2]

Panics about sexual crime are nothing new. History is littered with examples of periods when the public is obsessed by the notion that they, or their children, are at risk of sexual assault. Fifteenth-century Dijon saw a series of gang-rapes involving, on one estimate, half of the young males in the city and leading to high levels of anti-rape hysteria.[3] In the eighteenth century, the

European aristocracy was swept with a wave of hysteria about
the possibility that their children would be sexually molested by
chambermaids and nurses. So fearful was James Stuart, the Old
Pretender, that he rejected his wife's advice and employed a male
tutor, causing the break-up of his marriage and reducing his
chances of restoration.[4]

Such episodes should be treated with caution. Their occurrence is
often evidence of an underlying disquiet about the stability of
society: as Jeffrey Richards has shown,[5] sexual deviants have provided a ready source of scapegoats for the authorities at a time when
the social order is perceived to be under threat.

Richards argues that it has been common practice to level
accusations of sexual malpractice at outsiders of all sorts: the
derivation of the word 'bugger', for example, is a direct result of
the process of attributing vice to those who are seen as posing a
threat to the established social order. The Albigensian heretics of
the twelfth century became known in England as 'Bulgars' after
the country in which the Manichean heresy had originated.
Despite the fact that the Albigensian sect preached sexual abstin-
ence, they were frequently accused of homosexuality by a
Catholic Church anxious to denigrate them. So regularly was the
charge of homosexuality linked with the name Bulgar that the
two became inextricably linked in English.

There is therefore little new in the current panic about sexual
crime. The obsession of the press with stories of rape and sexual
abuse is nothing to the explosion in the newspaper coverage of
sexual crime in the 1840s and 1850s.[6] It is also intriguing to
compare the wilder claims about the phenomenon of satanic
sexual abuse with some of the charges laid against the door of
heretics in the Middle Ages: the linking of heterodoxy with devil
worship and child abuse goes back at least to the burning of a
group of ascetic Orleans friars in 1022, and echoes accusations
made by Roman propagandists against early Christians.

But sexual crime is a real phenomenon, and its victims real
women, children and men. It is difficult to read accounts by
survivors of sexual abuse without experiencing distress and deep
anger. But they are essential reading. Without them, it is all too
easy to underestimate the seriousness of many sexual crimes and
the suffering of victims. Many are unambiguous in their violence
and horror:

When I was young, he did a lot of things in front of the family: french kissing, fondling. Later on, it was regular intercourse. At age ten, the sex got more and more violent, and that's when I started to get hurt. It got more perverse. I don't know what he used – he had dental instruments – he put them inside me.[7]

We got to the flat and he dragged me into the bedroom and – oh I just wanted him to go, I wanted him to get out. Then he forced me into the bed, made me have sex with him and he scratched all my back open. Then he got a can of deodorant and sprayed it into every scratch then he started laughing and said 'Go and show that to your boyfriend'.[8]

Other accounts more readily expose the more subtle and collusive impact of abuse on victims:

And so I would lie in the bed, with him reading a story, and trying at the same time to put his hands in the bed, or putting his hands in the bed, and me lying with my legs crossed as tight as I could hold them, trying to fight it off – but ultimately having my clitoris manipulated so that it did start to turn me on, and always giving in and always coming. So I was caught in that total dilemma of 'I don't want this to happen' and then 'I do want it', over and over again, and trying to fight it off, and getting into it.[9]

The current panic about sexual crime, then, is grounded in a real truth. Sexual crime leaves women, children and men with psychological and physical scars which may never heal. The threat posed by sexual offenders also appears to be growing. The official statistics reveal a steady pattern: there is, it seems, an inexorable rise in the number of sexual offences being committed. Fear of sexual crime is increasing: the British Crime survey found that the number of women reporting their fear of being the victim of sexual attack increased from 23 per cent in 1982 to 30 per cent in 1984.[10]

It is to our criminal justice system that the public looks for a response to the threat of sexual crime. The police, the courts, the probation service and the prison service: these are the agencies whose policies towards the increasing number of sex offenders entering the system will crucially affect the future not just of those offenders but also the behaviour of other offenders and hence victims. This book is an attempt to examine how the policies of these agencies have been affected by the panic about sexual crime. It examines the current explanations for sexual abuse and the number of offences being committed. It looks at sentencing policy and the role of the probation and prison services. And it asks how far the policies of the penal system have proved a rational and sensible response to the phenomenon of sexual crime.

Chapter 1

Background to the phenomenon: definitions and explanations

The starting point for any investigation into the penal response to sexual offending must be the theoretical background to the phenomenon. Three questions must be answered. What do we mean by sexual offending? What causes individuals to commit sexual offences? And are such offenders amenable to treatment?

Posing these questions immediately risks being embroiled in heated academic debate. Definitions and explanations of sexual crime are the focus for acrimonious discussion among psychologists, biologists and sociologists, and the differing academic and political perspectives from which they approach the problem often appear to render any meaningful and balanced debate impossible.

This is not just an academic argument, but one crucial to any critique of penal policy. Attempts to assess the true level of sexual crime require some agreement on those acts that are to be defined as sexual offences. Questions about the causes of offending and the treatability of offenders have a direct impact on the proper policy of courts towards sexual offenders and on the proper role of the prisons and probation service. Indeed, it is arguable that it is because these questions have not been carefully examined that recent penal policy towards sex offenders has been so disjointed.

BASIC DEFINITIONS

The first question is: What do we mean by a sexual offence? Superficially, the answer is obvious. The term 'sex offending' denotes those activities involving sex which are deemed to be outside the law. However, the law relating to sexual behaviour is often confused. For many years the precise legal status of rape within marriage has been a matter for considerable debate. In

England, the Chief Justice Hale judgement of 1736, which held that a woman gave her body and consent to sex as part of the marriage contract, was only overturned by the House of Lords on 23 October 1991. Even then, the Law Lords were adamant that legislation is needed to clarify the situation.

This confusion also besets other sexual activity. The legal status of sado-masochism was thrown into doubt by a House of Lords ruling in a recent case involving a homosexual sado-masochistic sex ring, which held that the men concerned could be convicted of committing assaults on each other, despite the fact that what took place was with the full consent of all the partici-pants. An even more curious twist was added when some defendants pleaded guilty to aiding and abetting assaults upon themselves.[1] Even where the law is clear, there are obvious ano-malies. Consensual buggery between males over 21 in private is legal; consensual buggery of a woman by a man is not.[2]

There is also little agreement about what is to be classified as a 'sexual' crime. English law, unlike that of many other jurisdic-tions, makes no formal distinction between sexual and non-sexual offending. The nearest thing we possess to a formal list of sexual offences comes in the Sexual Offences Act 1956, which forms the basis of the official Home Office statistics. These classify sexual crime into twelve separate classes of notifiable offence: buggery, indecent assault on a male, indecency between males, rape, indecent assault on a female, unlawful sexual inter-course (USI) with a girl under 13, USI with a girl under 16, incest, procuration, abduction, bigamy, and gross indecency with a child. When official statistics of the extent of sexual crime are issued, these are the crimes which are being counted.

The list covers a wide range of human behaviours. One amended version details forty-three different criminal offences involving sex. As a number of the provisions create more than one offence, the total number of different sexual offences possible runs into several hundred. However, these behaviours appear to have in little in common apart from a connection with sex. The list mixes together offences which require the performance of sexual acts (buggery, rape), offences which are motivated by sex but where no sexual act has actually taken place (abduction), and offences which are less directly sex-related (bigamy, procura-tion). Some acts, such as flagellation, are illegal by virtue of the act; others, such as rape, because of the lack of consent. Some acts, such as bestiality, are illegal by nature of the identity of the victim; in some, age is a vital variable – sexual intercourse is legal between a man of 20 and a girl of 16 if the latter consents but not if the girl is 15. Others depend merely upon the location – consenting homosexual sex between males over 21 is legal in private but not in public places.

Such a confused list scarcely provides a coherent definition of sexual crime. On the one hand, it includes offences which appear to bear little relation to sex. A Howard League Working Party on unlawful sex suggested that the classification of bigamy as a sexual offence was an outdated anomaly, and that it should be omitted. The position of other offences, such as those connected with prostitution, was more complicated, the Working Party argued. Although they are classified in Home Office Criminal Statistics as 'sexual' and contain crucial sexual elements, in many ways they have more to do with economic necessity than with sex.[3]

At the same time, the Home Office list excludes many offences which may contain a crucial sexual element. Indecent exposure is not formally classified as a sexual offence. Cases of aggravated burglary, a charge often used where a sexual assault has taken place during the course of a break-in, do not appear in official statistics as sexual crimes. The rape of a woman followed by her murder would be classified in the statistics as a crime of violence rather than as a sexual offence.

There is also the question of how far we should broaden or narrow our definition of which aspects of sexual behaviour should be classified as crimes. Andrea Dworkin has called for all sexual activity 'not initiated by women' to be classed as rape.[4] It has also been argued that serial murders of women, such as those committed by Peter Sutcliffe, where no actual sexual assault took place, should be considered as sexual.[5]

However, many would argue that the Home Office list contains 'crimes' without victims, and that its range should be reduced rather than broadened. During the passage of the 1991 Criminal Justice Act, the gay activist organizations Outrage and the Stonewall Group argued vigorously against consenting homosexual activities between adult males being classified as sexual offences. In the initial drafting of the Bill, offences such as soliciting and indecency fell under the provisions of Section 25 of the Act, allowing sentencers to pass sentences of preventative detention on repeat offenders. However, this Section of the Act was not to be applied to offences involving (heterosexual) prostitution.[6] These groups argued instead that the age of consent in the case of homosexual sex should be lowered to match that in the case of heterosexual sex. Males engaging in sex with other males over the age of 16 should not be classified as 'sex offenders', with all the opprobrium that implies. Still less should there be any search for an explanation for their behaviour or attempts at 'treatment'.

These arguments enjoy powerful support. The Labour Party is committed to a lowering of the age of consent for homosexual sex to 16. The European Commission is also reported to be examining ways of standardizing ages of consent within the European Community.[7] This process could well cause problems, even for the Labour Party. The age of consent is frequently lower elsewhere in Europe than it is in the UK: in Italy, the age of consent for both hetero- and homosexual sex is 14, in Spain 12.[8]

Some would take matters further. The magazine *Understanding Paedophilia*, published by the Paedophile Information Exchange, carried articles advocating the complete abandonment of the concept of a legal age of consent, citing historical and foreign examples of the occurrence and acceptance of sex between adults and children. These contacts it regarded as healthy, positive and normal. It is only when there is 'the use of threats, violence, unreasonable coercion, drugs, etc.' that the law should intervene.[9] Otherwise, paedophile sexual activity is natural, normal and requires no explanation.

Such claims go to the heart of the debate about what constitutes sexual crime. Despite (or indeed because of) the anger and disgust these arguments arouse, coherent attempts to counter them have been relatively rare.[10] The traditional reliance on appeals to simple concepts of 'normality' and 'morality' as the basis for determining what should, and what should not, be classified as sexual crime has little force. Paedophilia, homosexuality and incest have been relatively common in both ancient and contemporary societies. Even within Christian Western society, the degree of moral turpitude attached to such acts as buggery and masturbation has varied according to the needs and attitudes of the time.[11]

The touchstones of normality and morality therefore appear of little use. However, that does not mean that no meaningful distinctions about what constitutes (or should constitute) sexual crime can be made. There is a basic distinction that can be drawn between sex which is deviant or illegal and sexual abuse, between behaviour which produces victims and behaviour which does not. Unless a sexual act is freely entered into with full, informed consent, or if its consequences are seriously harmful, then, it can be argued, it should be classified as a sexual crime. Thus rape and all non-consensual sex are sexual abuse, but consensual, non-exploitative homosexual activity is not.

Many abusers, however, would defend their behaviour even in the face of such a distinction. Many rapists would argue that their victim enjoyed the experience. The central tenet of paedophile faith is that sex between adults and children is not harmful, and that it is freely entered into and fully consensual. There is some research evidence to support the paedophile case. Sandford found in his study of paedophile sex that many of the children reported it as a positive and pleasurable experience.[12] Similar findings have been reported in the case of incest.[13]

However, the weight of evidence is overwhelming in rejecting the abusers' arguments. The testimony of survivors quoted in the introduction is scarcely consistent with abusers' claims. As Finkelhor points out (and confirms by means of data from his own surveys), the overwhelming majority of children who have had sexual experiences with adults do not regard it as having been a positive experience.[14] Moreover, the research on the impact of abuse upon survivors' lives is often devastating. The experience of abuse has been linked with later psychiatric problems, with the use of drugs, homelessness and prostitution.[15] There is also some evidence that survivors of abuse experience later sexual problems.[16]

Nor can the claims made by abusers, that victims often consented, be allowed to pass unchallenged. The testimony of rape survivors repeatedly bears out the fact that when verbal consent is given, it is invariably under the threat of violence or coercion. The thesis that children freely consent to sexual involvement with adults is also questionable. Not only is it the case that what is presented as free consent on the part of the child is often unwilling consent elicited by threats and manipulation. It is also misleading to claim that children can give genuine consent to an activity about which they are often very ignorant, when they may not yet have developed the emotional maturity to deal with the experience.

The distinction between sexual abuse and non-abusive illegal sex is fundamental to the operation of the criminal justice response to sexual offending. It provides a justification for the intervention of the legal system in sex between adults and chidren (or older children and younger children). However, this justification becomes weaker as the children involved become older, with a consequent advance in knowledge and emotional maturity. It is also weaker in cases of apparently consensual under-age sex between children of the same age, where the dangers of abuse of power and authority are not so palpable, and which is not linked with such problematic after-effects. Indeed, it appears from the Kinsey Report and other surveys that, for most people, their first sexual experiences are as children with other children.[17] Although, in theory, the ubiquity of under-age sexual experience puts the majority of the British population into the category of 'sex offender', in practice the operation of the law observes the distinction between sexual abuse and illegal sex, and rarely if ever intervenes.

Limiting one's definition of sexual crime to abusive sex has crucial advantages in the search for an explanation of its cause. The huge range of behaviours that can be defined as sexual offending would otherwise make such a search impossible. Given the range of offences and the different nature of the circum- stances that render them illegal, the search for explanation would appear not simply difficult but prima facie illogical. The violent rape of a stranger seems to have little in common with consensual homosexual sex in a public convenience, and an incident involv- ing a middle-aged adult buggering a 5-year-old boy appears to differ fundamentally from the case of two 15-year-olds having consensual heterosexual intercourse. Although all four cases involve the commission of sexual acts which are against the law, it is difficult to see any other common feature.

EXPLANATIONS

It is for this reason that few of the explanations that are advanced for sexual crime seek to explain the full range of sexual behaviours that may fall foul of the law. Instead, they concentrate almost exclusively on sexual assaults against women and children. The most recent attempts to explain these fall broadly into three schools: the sociological, the biological, and the psycho- logical. The first explains the occurrence of sexual crime (especi- ally rape) by the operation of power and gender relationships in society, the second by Darwinian theories of evolution or by the influence of hormones on behaviour, and the third by the psychological functioning of individual offenders.

However, before moving on to consider the precise nature of those theories, three caveats need to be added about the research on which they are based. First, as the next chapter will show, very little sexual crime ever comes to the attention of the authorities, let alone in a form that is capable of being studied by criminologists or psychologists. Conclusions based on in-depth studies of convicted sexual offenders, or even on interviews with survivors of sexual abuse, are therefore undermined by the unrepresentative nature of their samples. As the authors of a recent study of convicted and imprisoned rapists admit:

> It should be emphasised at this stage that the present study has looked at a population composed entirely of men who have been both convicted of and imprisoned for rape. Any generalisations about rapists who are not in prison, either because they have not been reported, apprehended, or convicted, should be made with extreme caution, if at all.[18]

The second caveat is about the reliability of interviews with offenders themselves. There is considerable evidence to indicate that sex offenders are more than usually reluctant to provide accurate accounts of their offending. In the study quoted above, Grubin and Gunn found that only 41 per cent of the interviewed rapists were willing to admit that their convictions were correct. This is consistent with other research into the extent of denial among sexual offenders.[19] Those offenders who were prepared to give full and accurate accounts of their offences clearly form an even more unrepresentative sample, and what they say should be treated with considerable caution.

If these difficulties were not enough, for those working in the British penal system, there is another problem. There has been relatively little research into sexual offending in a British context. The vast majority of the published research is from the USA or Canada. While much of this research is extremely useful, one should hesitate before adopting it as being valid for Britain too. Rates of reported sexual crime, and evidence about the underlying rate of crime, tend to indicate that there are considerable differences in its incidence between the USA, Canada and Britain. There are also important legal differences between the differing jurisdictions. Thus, for example, oral sex is illegal in some states in the USA, as the British lawyer Clive Stafford-Smith discovered when he came across a man in a Georgia prison serving five years for consensual oral sex with his wife.[20] There may well also be cultural differences (about, for example, attitudes to women and children, or the availability of pornography, drugs, or alcohol) which crucially affect the nature of sexual offending.

None of these difficulties suggests that research into the nature of sexual offending should be discarded completely. Nevertheless, such research should be treated with caution. It is not always clear what definitions of sexual crime are being used or how the offenders or offences under study have been selected. Interview techniques differ wildly from the unstructured to the structured, from the passive to the strongly guided; as a consequence, it is often difficult to deduce whether what is recorded is the unchallenged view of the offender, replete with half-truths and self-justifications, or the theoretical perspective of the interviewer imposed upon the account of the offender or victim. Follow-up times for treated offenders are often far too short, and different definitions of failure of treatment are used. Studies are therefore rarely directly comparable, and conclusions can only be tentatively held.

SOCIOLOGICAL THEORY

The first explanation to be considered is the sociological theory of sexual abuse. This theory, grounded in a feminist analysis of society, was most powerfully articulated by Susan Brownmiller in her book *Against Our Will*.[21] Brownmiller and her followers argue that rape and sexual abuse of women and children is an inevitable product of a society in which men dominate political and economic life. A society which denies women and children power render them unequal partners in decision making. Their opinions come to count for little, and their wishes can be overridden by men. Male myths flourish: 'no doesn't really mean no'; 'all women fantasize about rape'; 'they enjoy it really'. Prostitution and pornography, in which women are forced to participate out of economic necessity, only reinforce this view by portraying them solely in terms of their availability for men's sexual desire. The result is that men become educated to think of women and children as property, as objects for their sexual gratification, whose consent to sex is not important. Indeed, the early Western legal definitions of rape were in terms of a crime against property: the rape of a married woman was not a crime against the woman herself but against her husband or father. The power imbalance in society renders rape inevitable.

But Brownmiller and some supporters of this thesis go further. Rape, they argue, is not simply the result of women's subservience to men, but a strategy engaged in by men to keep women subservient. Rape, and the threat of rape, serves to reduce women's participation in society and therefore their opportunity to challenge men's dominance. Brownmiller states this view unambiguously:

> From prehistorical times to the present, I believe, rape has played a critical function: it is nothing more or less than a conscious process of intimidation by which *all* men keep *all* women in a state of fear.[22]

On this view of rape and sexual abuse, the motivation for the act is not necessarily, or even essentially, sexual. Rape is instead a 'pseudosexual act', its motivation dominance, even anger.[23] Hence the use of rape to humiliate women who threaten the established order: in 1991, Farhana Hayat was gang-raped in Pakistan, a rape allegedly carried out by secret police on the orders of a Pakistani Home Office Minister because of her friendship with the opposition leader Benazir Bhutto.[24]

This characterization of rape as a pseudosexual act finds striking parallels in writings about male rape. Rape and abuse of men by other men has received relatively little attention, despite the indications that it is far more common than might be otherwise supposed.[25] The few published studies tend to indicate that sexual abuse of men is rarely motivated by sexual desire. It is usually carried out by men who regard themselves as heterosexual and who claim that they would never engage in consensual homosexual acts.[26] The primary motivation is to humiliate. A striking example of this came at the inquest of Lee Waite, who committed suicide in Feltham Young Offenders Institution in August 1991 because of bullying, when it was revealed that other prisoners had pushed a snooker cue into his rectum.[27]

There is considerable evidence to support the feminist view of sexual offending. The hypothesis that a willingness to engage in rape and sexual assault is not confined to a small group of 'abnormal' men has been confirmed by surveys which indicate that rape and sexual assault are relatively widespread and accepted behaviours in Western society. One study found that 44 per cent of male American college students reported some likelihood that they would rape,[28] another that 35 per cent of men would rape if they thought they would not get caught.[29] Similar studies have also indicated a correlation between belief in rape myths and aggression against women.[30]

However, although the analysis is a compelling one and has established itself as the most influential contemporary explanation of sexual crime, it is not without its weaknesses. The hypothesis that sexual assault is the inevitable consequence of the inequality in power relationships between the genders has some support: some cross-cultural analyses have found a correlation between the sharing of power between the genders and a low incidence of rape.[31] There are nevertheless obvious counterexamples: women in Japan appear to enjoy less power than women in many Western societies, but the (apparent) rates of rape and sexual assault are higher in the West.

Supporters of the thesis could explain this difficulty by arguing that high Western rates of rape are the result of men feeling threatened by women's gains in power and status. However, the belief that rape is part of a 'conscious process of intimidation' and is motivated primarily by anger is difficult to accept as an explanation for all, or even most, rapes. The phenomenon of 'date-rape', which, according to victim surveys, accounts for a sizeable proportion of rapes, appears an obvious exception to this pattern. Although offenders might be angry at having their sexual advances rejected, sexual desire is clearly fundamental. Only a small minority of date-rapists report that the motivation for their offence was domination.[32] In most cases, rapists describe their offences in sexual terms and aspire to what they regard as successful sexual performance during the act.[33]

The theory is also unable to explain the diverse patterns of human sexual desire. By itself, the feminist theory struggles to explain the fact that some men are sexually aroused primarily by children or other men. Nor is it able to deal with the (comparatively rare) examples of sexual offending by women, except where women have been forced into offending by male threats or coercion. The constant equating of sexual assaults with male power seems at odds with examples of females using positions of power to abuse.[34]

BIOLOGICAL THEORIES

Like the sociological theory, the Darwinian version of the biological theory sees rape and sexual abuse primarily as products of
societal functioning, rather than of individual pathology. Like
Brownmiller and her successors, its proponents argue that all
men have the built-in potential to rape a woman. However, the
biologists argue that this potential springs not from the nature of
the power relationships between the genders but from the biological imperative of evolution.

The Darwinian version of the biological theory seeks principally
to explain the occurrence of rape. However, its proponents maintain
that it is only a matter of time before it can be expanded to cover
child abuse (and homosexuality).[35] Simply stated, the theory argues
that human sexual behaviour, like that of any animal, is driven by
the need for humans to attempt to maximize their potential for
successful reproduction. There is therefore a difference between the
needs of males and females. The interests of a female lies in the
successful attraction of a mate who will be able to care for and
support her and her offspring after mating. For males, the successful
strategy is one which maximizes the opportunity for reproduction:
the successful male is the one who impregnates a large number of
fertile females. Rape is therefore to be seen as a mating strategy
entered into by relatively unsuccessful males. Unable to attract
females because they do not possess the characteristics which indicate that they can provide care and support for mother and offspring,
they are forced to engage in rape in order to have any chance of
reproduction. For the biologists, rape is primarily about reproduction.

Unsurprisingly, this view of rape has not been universally
endorsed. Nevertheless, its proponents have some evidence to
support it. It is true that it is women around the peak ages of
reproduction who are most likely to be raped, as the theory
would predict.[36] Most (albeit not all) rapists are poor, ill-
educated, and relatively powerless; it can be argued that they are
therefore relatively less likely than other men to be able to attract
a mate.[37] There is also some evidence to indicate that, in some
cases, rape is a successful strategy for men to gain continued
reproductive access to a female partner. According to Russell,[38]
some victims of rape become bound to their attacker by 'trauma-
induced bonding and dependency' and a continuing relationship develops. Some even marry the man who raped them.

However, there are greater reasons to be suspicious of the theory. First, and despite the claims of its proponents to scientific rigour, the scientific basis of the theory remains unproven. Attempts to derive general evolutionary theories from the observation of the behaviour of insects and animals, and to apply them to a complex set of behaviours such as human reproductive strategies remain controversial within the scientific community. Nor does an appeal to the role of genetic influence to explain differing rates of rape around the world succeed in the absence of any indications that any genes or combination of genes exist to explain behaviours as complex as rape.

Equally questionable is the view of rape as a reproductive strategy. While it may be true that the majority of victims are at peak reproductive age, it is equally true that girls below the age of puberty and women past child-bearing age are also the victims of rape. Some studies have found that some rapists are not particularly concerned as to the gender of their victim.[39] Although rape does clearly carry some likelihood of the impregnation of the victim, there are also indications that in only about half of all rapes does the rapist actually ejaculate, and many of the sexual acts commonly entered into by rapists, such as oral sex and buggery,[40] could not result directly in impregnation. In approximately one-third of reported cases, rapists also inflict gratuitous violence on their victims and, in a significant number of cases, rape is followed by murder.[41] The explanation that

> . . . severe injury or death caused by a rape offender, as well as much of the variance in offender behaviour unexplained by our evolutionary hypothesis (e.g. rape of pre- or post-reproductive women) can be attributed to accident or psychotic mentality[42]

is inadequate. There is little to indicate that rapists are any more likely to suffer from psychiatric problems than other offenders.[43] It is also difficult to believe that the levels of serious violence done to women in the course of rapes can be accounted for by accidents.

This version of the biological theory is strictly limited. It does not seek to explain the sexual abuse of women that stops short of rape and the sexual abuse of other men and of children. It is difficult to see how such abuse can be explained in terms of a theory which argues that humans are driven by the need to reproduce. Although this does not in itself undermine the arguments adduced by the biologists to explain rape, their failure to explain any other types of sexual behaviour is perhaps significant.

The hormonal version of the biological school has more to recommend it. The possibility that hormonal imbalances may influence offenders to abuse has been the subject of increasing interest in recent years. Research has concentrated on the links between sex and aggression, which appear to be mediated by the neural substrates and activated by the same endocrines, the sex steroids.[44] There is some evidence that a higher than normal proportion of particularly aggressive or sadistic rapists have high sex steroid levels.[45] However, there is little to indicate that this is true of a substantial proportion of abusers. It seems simply as though many sex offenders have failed to learn to control the increases in sex steroid levels associated with puberty.

PSYCHOLOGICAL THEORIES

Both the sociological and the Darwinian version of the biological theory advance explanations for the phenomenon of sexual abuse. However, neither provides much in the way of guidance about why an individual offender abuses. For such explanations, unless one accepts the hormonal version of the biological theory, one must turn to theories grounded in individual psychology. These are particularly attractive because they often bring with them the promise of enabling the reform of the individual offender. However, there is little agreement between the competing schools of psychology, and some of the theories have almost no empirical evidence to support them.

Psychological explanations of sexual offending have been slow to develop. For a long time there was little attempt by psychoanalytic theorists – until recently the dominant force in forensic psychology – to address the issue of sexual offending, largely because of Freud's belief that accounts of childhood sexual abuse were fantasy, and because of the confusion in his writings between rape and seduction.[46] The prevailing explanation of sexual crime characterized abusers as inadequate, immature or mentally disordered, abusing through drunkenness or because of some action on the part of the offended which had aroused uncontrollable impulses in the offender. This is certainly still the popular image: in a survey conducted for *Company* magazine, over half of the respondents believed that men who attack women were 'usually socially or sexually inadequate', and many thought that they were 'pathetic failures who could only feel achievement by dominating others'.[47] It is, arguably, still the view of some judges.

It is a view which has some evidence to support it. There are some indications that sexual abusers have poor impulse control and there is considerable evidence to show a link between alcohol use and sexual offending.[48] There is also support for the explanation that some sexual offenders are inadequate, are emotionally immature, or lack social skills;[49] it can be argued that they offend because their inadequacies or lack of social skills deny them easy access to legal sexual relations.

However, this evidence is strictly limited. There is little to indicate that sexual offenders are any more likely than other offenders to have had a history of mental disorder: the traditional explanation that old men who abuse children must be senile appears to have no foundation. Moreover, there are dangers in drawing easy conclusions from statistical correlations. Evidence that many (if not most) sexual offenders have consumed alcohol before committing their offences only indicates that alcohol may frequently be used by offenders as a deliberate disinhibiter.

It is also perhaps significant that these explanations appear to remove from offenders the responsibility for their actions. As Bart and O'Brien have pointed out:

> It is interesting, if not suspicious, that each of these supposed psychological causes is put in the kind of legal language that can be used in court to defend the assailant so that he may be found not guilty.[50]

More recently, cognitive/behavioural explanations of sexual offending have come to dominate. The cognitive/behavioural theory of writers such as Bandura argues that sexually abusive behaviour is behaviour that is, or can be, learned.[51] Sexual offenders come to associate certain stimuli – be they scenes of violence against women or images of children – with sexual satisfaction, perhaps as the result of a childhood sexual experience. This sexual orientation is reinforced by masturbation to fantasies of rape or child abuse. It is also sustained by belief systems designed to justify and support abusive behaviour: that children can consent to and enjoy sex; that sex between children and adults is natural and healthy; that women enjoy rape, and that when a woman says no it sometimes (or always) means yes. These beliefs are derived in part from contact with other offenders with similar beliefs in locations such as prisons. However, they are also derived from the attitude of broader society: societal attitudes to women, it is argued, reinforce the beliefs of rapists and the availability of child pornography has been linked to child sexual abuse.[52] These belief systems have the added advantage for offenders of serving to justify their behaviour and minimize any guilt that they might feel.

This theory has taken particular force from indications that many abusers claim they were themselves victims of abuse. Groth and Burgess[53] found that 32 per cent of a sample of convicted sexual offenders reported having been the victims of abuse when they were younger; in comparison, only 3 per cent of a sample of police officers reported abuse. There is evidence of intergenerational transmission of incest.[54] The Grubin and Gunn survey of convicted rapists also found that 20 per cent of their sample reported having been abused when they were children – in 11 per cent of cases on a regular basis. Victims become abusers, creating more victims and more abusers. This 'cycle of abuse' not merely provides an explanation for sexual offending, it also provides campaigners for greater public awareness of child sexual abuse with a powerful argument to justify engaging in work with victims and offenders alike.

However, the fact that many sexual offenders report experience of sexual abuse (or extensive early sexual experience) does not necessarily show a causal link with their later offending. Other factors may be involved. Grubin and Gunn reported that there was a strong association between their rapists' reports of sexual abuse and their reports of other physical abuse and that it was impossible to conclude whether sexual abuse was a significant factor in their offending.[55] The tendency of abusers to report childhood abuse and link that to their behaviour may only be a method of explaining their offences and minimizing their guilt. Finally, while there are a large number of victims of sexual abuse, most of whom are female, there appear to be far fewer abusers, most of whom are male. It is difficult to explain this in terms of a causal link between being abused and becoming an abuser. Some victims of sexual abuse may take on the identity and behaviour of a sexual abuser, but the process of learning how to become an abuser requires more than just exposure to abuse.

Nevertheless, this analysis of how abusive behaviour progresses and is reinforced is a compelling one. It can go some way towards explaining why individual offenders are sexually attracted to children, for example, and why some (but by no means all) offenders move from one form of sexual offending (for example, flashing) towards more serious form (such as rape). It draws strength from the fact that it is rooted in empirical psychology and that its analysis of the belief systems that sustain and reinforce offending has much in common with the feminist analysis of sex offending. Perhaps, more importantly, it holds out an enticing promise that abusive behaviour can be changed: what has been learned can be unlearned.

INTEGRATED THEORIES

These various theories about the nature of sexual offending – structural explanations rooted in a feminist analysis of a patriarchal society or a biological analysis of human sexual behaviour, and psychological explanations rooted in analyses of the behaviour and characteristics of individual offenders – all have something to contribute to our understanding of sexual crime. However, they all have weaknesses, and each fails to deal adequately with the complex nature of abusive behaviour and the wide range of humans who become abusers.

These explanations are not mutually exclusive. In recent years, attempts have been made to produce integrated theories of sexual offending, combining elements from all three major schools. Two of these, Marshall and Barbaree's integrated theory of sexual abuse and Finkelhor's multi-factor analysis of abusive behaviour, now constitute the theoretical underpinning of almost all the work with sex offenders that is undertaken in the British penal system.

Marshall and Barbaree's integrated theory[56] takes as its starting point the principle that males have a biologically endowed propensity for pursuing their own sexual fulfilment, and a tendency to confuse sex and aggression. The task for males is to learn to control these tendencies. However, where individuals have been poorly socialised or exposed to destructive childhood experiences, they can become aggressive and insensitive to the needs and desires of others. Individuals who lack self-esteem learn to prove their masculinity through aggressive sex or abuse. Feelings of social inadequacy produce hostility towards others.

An individual's tendency towards abusing will also be crucially affected by sociological variables. Attitudes towards women and children, the norms of sexual behaviour, the availability of pornography, and the degree of tolerance shown by the wider society towards sexual abuse will all increase or decrease the likelihood that an offender will abuse. There are also more proximate factors which come into play. Many individuals will deliberately create opportunities to offend; others may be more reactive, responding to certain situations or stimuli, such as times of stress or anger, or when they are drunk, or when an opportunity to offend arises.

Finkelhor's analysis of sexual offending[57] is of a similar nature. It was originally devised as an explanation of child sexual abuse, but can easily be applied to abuse of adults too. It has four stages: motivation; overcoming internal inhibitors; overcoming external inhibitors; and overcoming the resistance of the victim. An offender must pass through all these stages if an offence is to take place.

First, offenders need to be motivated to become sexually involved with the victim. They may, for example, be sexually aroused by children, whether or not they are also aroused by adults. They may find scenes of rape sexually arousing. They may find that sexual involvement with children is more emotionally satisfying than involvement with adults. They may be inadequate, have poor social skills, or be in other circumstances where they feel that they are unable to achieve any consensual involvement with an adult. Any or all of these explanations may apply in any one case.

Second, offenders must overcome the factors which would inhibit their becoming sexually abusive. These inhibitors are of two sorts: internal and external belief systems which discourage rape or sexual involvement with children, and practical circumstances which prevent such involvement easily taking place. Offenders' own internal inhibitors, their moral scruples, can be bypassed by the use of alcohol, or may be weakened where offenders suffer from poor impulse control because of mental problems, psychosis, stress, or any other similar factors. The individual offender's overcoming of scruples may be assisted by wider social factors: the apparent toleration of sexual abuse, the myths supporting sexual offending, the availability of pornography, weak criminal sanctions, and a social ideology which encourages men to override the desires of women and children.

External inhibitors also need to be overcome for abuse to take place. Abuse can only take place if the abuser has access to the victim and the opportunity to abuse. In the case of incest, such opportunity may be easily secured. In the case of stranger rape or non-familial abuse, opportunities must be more actively sought. Some rapists plan their attacks. Many child abusers report that they deliberately plan opportunities to gain access to children: they seek out environments where children congregate, and cultivate acquaintance with people who have children. Many of those convicted of child abuse offended while working as teachers, scout leaders, and so on. It may be the case that such individuals offended not because they spent so much time with children that they eventually gave into temptation, but because they sought out positions with children so that they could offend.

Finally, the victim's resistance must be overcome. The fact that so many abusers are in positions of power or trust *vis-à-vis* their victim often enables the resistance to be overcome more easily. Threats, coercion, violence, bribery, and reward may all be used both for adults and children. Children may be easier to control: they may be isolated or deprived, ignorant of sexual matters, and may lack the knowledge or confidence to refuse. Offenders report 'grooming' their victims, and can become highly skilled in ensuring compliance and later silence.

Both analyses suggest that a variety of psychological and structural factors may have played a part in an individual sexual offence. If one accepts such an analysis, one has to accept too that there is no simple solution to sexual crime.

TREATMENT STRATEGIES

Since factors as different as the relative economic circumstances of men and women on the one hand, and the hormone levels of a particular offender on the other, may both play a part in causing an abuser to abuse, it is clearly impossible to guarantee that an offender can be successfully 'cured' of sexual offending. Were it the case that sexual offending had a simple cause, a simple solution could be found. But the range of phenomena that could play a part is so wide, and the difficulties of changing them so great, that even if a suitable 'treatment' could be devised for an individual offender, there could be no guarantee of its success.

That is not to say that nothing can be done to address factors that may have played a part in an individual's offences. Many of the explanations for sex offending bring with them their own manifestos for change. The sociological analysis of Brownmiller argues that sexual offending must be addressed through a radical reordering in society, an empowering of women and children and a coherent attempt to break down the patriarchal assumptions of men. Aspects of this manifesto have received support from proponents of the social learning theory, who have attacked the self-serving myths about women and children which reinforce offenders' behaviour, and have criticized the availability of (particularly child) pornography. Both theories emphasize treatment methods which involve challenging male attitudes towards women and children and myths about sexual crime. Discussing a recent visit to Grendon prison where over half of the prisoners have been convicted of sexual crime, Claire Glasman of Women against Rape concluded that:

> Most of the men were ready for an honest discussion . . . What the Grendon men said and their keenness to listen, bore out our conviction that men are not rapists by nature, and in the course of creating a society where women are economically and socially independent of men, we will see men change.[58]

However, for supporters of the integrated theories, this is only part of the answer. If abuse is the final act in a long chain of behaviours, attempts to change offenders' behaviour must begin with the analysis of the processes leading up to the act of abuse itself. In order to gain a realistic insight into the events which surrounded the offences and the feelings of the offenders, the first step is to break sex offenders' tendency towards denial. Researchers have repeatedly found that sex offenders minimize their part in their offences with a litany of excuses and myths. In particular, victims are blamed for encouraging the offender: they are said to be willing participants in the offence, and the offender is often presented as a passive 'victim' of what happened.[59] The true picture of events may only emerge after a considerable length of time.

Once the chain of behaviours which led to the offence has been laid bare, attempts can be made to teach offenders to interrupt it. The pattern of behaviour is analysed, and the offender's actions and feelings before and after each offence examined in detail. Here the analysis developed by Finkelhor is frequently used.

How offenders meet their victims, how they groom them, how they create the opportunity for their offences, how they overcome their own inhibitors and their victims' resistance – all these can be examined and strategies developed to enable offenders to interrupt their patterns of behaviour.

Many cognitive/behavioural theorists believe that the offender's initial stimulus to offend, the sexual orientation towards children as objects of sexual desire or rape as an arousing sexual image, can also be changed. This can be done by various means. For example, by the process of 'orgasmic reconditioning' offenders can be taught to substitute an acceptable sexual fantasy for the abusive fantasy to which they have been masturbating and which has reinforced their unacceptable sexual orientation through the pleasure of orgasm. The repeated coincidence of acceptable fantasy or image with the pleasure of orgasm, it is argued, helps offenders reorientate their pattern of sexual arousal. Similar techniques would teach offenders to interrupt their favourite abusive fantasies with distasteful or frightening images. Orgasmic reconditioning can be used to counter almost any pattern of arousal: one newspaper recently reported its successful use in dealing with a young man sexually obsessed with his parents' Austin Metro.[60]

Different techniques can be used to counter some of the other factors which may have contributed to a person's offending. If, for example, one factor in a particular person's offending is that he lacks sufficient social skills to be able easily to manage adult relationships, social skills training may be of use.[61] Many of these treatment methods can be used in group settings, and groupwork is seen as a particularly fruitful setting for encouraging offenders to admit the true nature of their offending. In particular, other sex offenders are often far more effective at breaking down their peers' systems of denial than are non-sex offenders.

Such treatment methods for sexual offenders now dominate the British penal scene: Leah Warwick found that most of the work with sex offenders being carried out in the probation service was derived from Finkelhor[62] and Marshall and Barbaree's analysis forms the basis for the treatment programme being introduced into twenty prisons in England and Wales. However, two other schools of treatment exist.

First, despite the difficulties posed by Freud's view of sexual abuse, psychodynamic treatment methods are used by many psychiatrists, probation officers and others working in the penal system. Psychodynamic methods revolve around the principle that aberrant sexual behaviour is a symptom of deeper, more fundamental problems, usually as a result of childhood trauma. Unless those problems are exposed and resolved, one cannot reduce the likelihood of the abusive behaviour recurring. These 'insight'-based treatments, usually undertaken on a one-to-one basis, often take as their focus an exploration of early childhood sexual adventures or traumas, rather than focusing specifically on the offences themselves.[63]

Second, programmes which rely upon the use of chemical treatments for sexual offending, including chemical castration, still have powerful proponents. Such programmes have as their basic assumption that many offenders have poor impulse control because of chemical imbalances in their system, and that the use of hormone-depressing chemicals can lower offenders' libido sufficiently to achieve a significant reduction in the likelihood of their commiting sexual offences. These have been used infrequently in the British penal system, not least because of the ethical difficulties involved: in 1987 the Mental Health Act Commission attempted to prevent one offender, Mark Witham, from receiving injections of goserelin, which left him 'with no sexuality whatever'; after taking his case to the High Court, Mr Witham was allowed to resume his treatment.[64] Similar worries about a Broadmoor doctor's use of libido-reducing implants formed the basis of a Channel 4 documentary.[65]

As has been argued above, there is little evidence to support the thesis that poor impulse control or abnormally high levels of testosterone occur in significant numbers of the sexual offenders who have been caught and convicted. Nor is there much research evidence to link testosterone levels with frequency of sexual activity.[66] It seems unlikely, therefore, that such treatments would benefit more than a small proportion of offenders, if indeed there is any direct benefit. Moreover, in merely depressing offenders' libido, chemical treatments would do nothing to change individuals' commitment to, say, a paedophilic orientation, or prevent them continuing to engage in sexual acts with children. The mere fact of reducing offenders' ability to produce an erection does not by itself prevent sexual offending.[67] Nevertheless, drug treatments may prove to be of use with individual offenders as part of a package of treatment.

The effectiveness of these various forms of treatment will be discussed in the concluding chapter. However, it is essential to note here that the doubts and confusions which beset the various explanations for the occurrence of sexual crime apply equally to the different schools of treatment. Just as our knowledge of the causes of sexual crime is patchy, so is our knowledge of the solutions to it.

Chapter 2

From crime to conviction

If the reason why offenders abuse is a matter for controversy, so is the frequency of abuse. Estimates of prevalence can vary wildly: some estimates put the proportion of children who suffer sexual abuse as high as 54 per cent,[1] others as low as 3 per cent.[2] The percentage of adult women who have been sexually attacked has been variously put at 37 per cent[3] and at only 10 per cent.[4] Even the question of whether more or fewer sexual offences are now being committed is a matter for debate.

This uncertainty would come as a considerable surprise to the general public. In the public mind, there is no doubt that the rate of sexual crime is increasing. Surveys of the public perception of crime have repeatedly shown that people believe that they are under an increasing threat from sexual crime.[5] This belief is apparently confirmed in the official statistics. The last few years have seen a significant increase in the officially recorded level of sexual crime as Table 2.1 shows.

These figures appear to reflect a marked growth in sexual crime over the 1980s. The total number of sexual offences recorded by the police has increased by 38 per cent, from 21,107 to 29,044. That rise compares with a rise in the general crime rate of 53 per cent over the same period, and a rise in all crimes of violence of 77 per cent. However, the increase in the number of recorded sexual offences has not been across the board. The number of offences of rape recorded has more than doubled, from 1,225 in 1980 to 2,498 in 1990, and this has been echoed by a rise in the number of offences of indecent assault on a female. On the other hand, the number of offences of unlawful sexual intercourse with a girl under 16 has declined by 31 per cent, and the number of cases of indecency between males by 18 per cent.

Table 2.1 Official statistics: notifiable sexual offences recorded by the police 1980–1990

	1980	*1985*	*1989*	*1990*
Buggery	657	633	1,138	1,120
Indecent assault on a male	2,288	2,307	2,878	3,043
Indecency between males	1,421	865	2,022	1,159
Rape	1,225	1,842	3,305	2,498
Indecent assault on a female	11,498	11,410	15,376	15,783
Unlawful sexual intercourse with a girl under 13	254	299	300	304
USI with a girl under 16	3,109	2,733	2,471	2,140
Incest	312	277	471	435
Procuration	104	229	113	176
Abduction	95	160	298	356
Bigamy	144	76	82	74
Gross indecency	*	633	1,279	1,063
Total	21,107	21,456	29,733	29,044[†]

*Figures not available prior to 1983.
† *Source*: *Criminal Statistics for England and Wales 1990* (London: HMSO, 1991).

However, there are good reasons to believe that these statistics are an inadequate guide to the true level of sexual crime. It is generally accepted that there is always some discrepancy between the rate of crime recorded in official statistics and the number of offences that are actually committed. That is hardly surprising. Many hurdles have to be successfully negotiated before a crime is recorded in the official crime statistics. An act has to take place and has to be identified by an individual as a crime. Someone has to decide to report the offence to the police, and be both motivated and able to do so. The police in turn have to believe that the act took place and they, too, have to classify the act as an offence. Finally, the police have to be sufficiently motivated to act on the report and record the fact that a crime has taken place.

The number and complexity of these stages allows consider-able scope for the process of a crime becoming an official statistic to break down. An act which is in contravention of the law may not be defined by participants or witnesses as criminal: fiddling of expenses, or shady dealings in the City, are good examples. Even when such an act is recognizably criminal, the intervention of the forces of law and order may be thought unnecessary or unwise. Many pub brawls are resolved without recourse to the police. Some offences – such as cases of minor theft – may not be reported because the chances of an arrest or conviction are not deemed high, or because the victim is too fearful to do so.

The attitude of the police is equally important. The conse-quences for a police officer accepting a crime report are con-siderable: forms have to be filled in and statements taken and typed. Valuable staffing time has to be devoted to following up the report. The police may be especially reluctant to do this when they believe that there is little chance of obtaining a conviction, or if the offence is deemed to be too trivial to warrant the time spent on it. A police officer may consider that what took place was not worth recording, or was even a crime.

For all these reasons, it is reasonable to assume that the official crime figures underestimate the true extent of offending. And if there are good reasons not to trust the official statistics relating to offences such as theft, those are redoubled in the case of sexual crime.

REPORTING RATES: OBSTACLES AND FEARS

To begin with, there are huge disincentives for those involved in sexual crime to report it to the police. Much sexual offending is either fully consensual or is not defined by its participants as a crime. Flagellation and heterosexual buggery are both against the law. Any sexual relationship under the age of 16 is illegal. Much homosexual activity takes place in breach of the law. Such acts would technically be sexual crimes, but would not be defined as such by the participants, and would certainly not be reported to the police. This may not always be a matter for much regret. It is of greater concern that some victims of child abuse may be too young to know that what is being done to them is illegal.

However, even sexual acts which are defined by participants or observers as crimes may still not be reported to the police. It is the low level of reporting of rape and sexual abuse which causes the greatest concern. This under-reporting happens for a variety of reasons. First, and most important, as interviews with abusers and victims have revealed, victims of sexual crime may be too fearful or too guilty to approach the authorities. Many offenders deliberately employ techniques of instilling guilt or fear in order to guarantee victims' silence. Victims are often traumatized by the experience of abuse and are made to feel complicit or responsible for it. So, for example, men who rape other men may masturbate their victims to ejaculation while buggering them; victims frequently take the fact that they have ejaculated as a sign that they must have enjoyed the experience, and their consequent feelings of confusion and shame militate against any decision to report.[6]

Similarly, child abusers often seek to engage the sympathy of the victim in order to set up a secret bond. Children are reminded of the harm that their revealing the abuse would do to the abuser, and the distress it would cause to others such as family members. They are told that no one will believe them if they do report the abuse, or that they would be taken away from their family; it has been reported that newspaper cuttings are shown to children to persuade them of this.[7] As La Fontaine has said: 'All authorities on the subject report that the pressure on victims to remain silent or to retract stories are heavy: threats of violence are not uncommon.'[8]

These techniques derive much of their effectiveness from the unequal power relationships between abuser and abused. Child abusers are often in positions of trust or responsibility over children: fathers, uncles, family friends, babysitters, teachers, older peers. These positions guarantee them access to their victims and the power to force them to participate in the abuse. They also provide the power, or threat of power, which can be used to ensure the children's silence. Similarly, a survey by Women Against Rape (WAR) revealed that 60 of the 145 rapes studied were committed by a husband, boyfriend, family member or man in authority.[9] Unsurprisingly, the fact that the rapist is known to the victim reduces the likelihood that the victims of rape will report the offence. In the WAR survey, none of the rapes committed by a husband or co-habitee was reported.[10] According to a survey by the London Rape Crisis Centre, half of the stranger rapes studied had been reported, but only one-quarter to one-fifth of attacks by a husband, boyfriend, or family member, and only one-fifth of attacks by a co-habitee.[11] Similar results have been reported from studies in Sweden.[12]

One reason for this is clearly economic. As the WAR study *Ask Any Woman* indicates, some women are trapped in relationships with violent and abusive men, and it is their lack of economic power to pursue suitable alternatives that condemns them to a toleration of the abuse.[13] Similar considerations may also be an important factor in children's decisions about whether or not to report. There may also be a fear about the reaction of family members, or even of the wider community:[14] the prosecution and conviction of a young man for sexually abusing a child led to attacks on the victim's home, and the victim and family were forced into hiding.[15]

These fears may ensure that many offences go unreported. Moreover, in the case of marital rapes, there was until recently literally no point in reporting the offence to the police. One recent survey estimated that one in seven married women has been raped by their present or previous husband, and in four out of five of these cases the offence had occurred more than once. Half of these rapes had been accompanied by the threat or use of violence, and one in five had taken place when the woman was pregnant.[16] However, until the ground-breaking House of Lords judgement in the case of *Regina v R.* in October 1991,[17] the rape of a wife by a husband was not illegal.

However, it was noticeable that the House of Lords judgement was received with considerable caution by both the police and some prominent legal experts. Although the Association of Chief Police Officers welcomed the ruling, police officials warned about the difficulty of proving cases of marital rape.[18] A spokesperson for the Crown Prosecution Service also emphasized that the CPS's own criteria require a reasonable prospect of a conviction before a prosecution can be undertaken.[19] It is doubtful whether such publicity will truly encourage women to take the step of reporting marital rape, or police to take such reports seriously.

Many offences may also go unreported because of the victims' fears about the response they will receive from the police. In the WAR study, 37 per cent of women who did not report the rape gave the fear that the police would not believe them as the major reason for not reporting; no less than 79 per cent of the non-reporters said that they feared the police would be unhelpful or unsympathetic.[20] In the past, these fears had considerable basis in truth, as police handling of victims of sexual offences has often been insensitive and ignorant.[21] Scenes such as the harsh interrogation of a rape victim shown in the BBC television documentary *Police* in January 1982 have only confirmed many women in the belief that their reception by the police will be traumatic in itself. Evidence from rape crisis centres and victims' support schemes indicated that such treatment was not unusual.[22]

Much of the evidence for poor police practice dates from the 1970s and there are indications that police handling of victims of sexual assault has subsequently improved. In 1986, the Home Office issued a circular 69/86 calling for new police training on rape and sexual assault, the appointment of new women police surgeons, and better facilities for examination. The police have recently admitted that their treatment of victims of sexual offences has been less than perfect,[23] and have taken initiatives, such as the establishment of 'rape suites' and specialist teams, to improve the service they offer. Dedicated rape suites are now to be found in over half the police force areas in the country,[24] and there is some evidence that victims who report the offences are now pleasantly surprised by their treatment by the police.[25] Public perceptions have yet to catch up with changes in police practice.

Victims are also fearful of what will happen to them in court. The rough handling of victims of rape by defence lawyers and judges has become notorious, and as with police practice, the advances that have been made in adapting judicial practice to the needs of victims of sexual crime have been too few and too late. In particular, concern has centred upon the roles of defence lawyers, judges and the media.

Cross-examination of the victim has been an area of particular worry. The primary responsibility of a defence lawyer is of course not towards the victim, but towards the defendant. Most sexual offences take place in private, and there are rarely any witnesses other than the victim. It is also rare that there is any supporting forensic evidence. The case, therefore, often rests upon the victim's word, and if the victim's testimony can be made to seem untrustworthy, then an acquittal is inevitable. The cross-examination of the victim is therefore often the centre of the trial.

Defence lawyers will use various techniques to break down the victim's testimony. The victim may be required to repeat the story of events in minute detail, with the lawyer probing for any inconsistencies; this may include requiring the victim to testify not only at the trial but also at a full committal hearing at a Magistrates' Court.[26] Where, at a rape trial, the issue is one of consent, attempts may be made to establish that the victim gave consent, or that consent was implied by the victim's behaviour, dress or past sexual behaviour. This may include detailed cross-examination of the victim's sexual history. Despite the restrictions placed on such cross-examination in the Sexual Offences (Amendment) Act 1976, questioning of victim's past sexual experience is still commonplace: one survey revealed that in only one-quarter of cases did judges refuse applications to raise the topic in questioning.[27] Protection is greater for child witnesses, but there are still indications that the experience of giving evidence at a trial is actively harmful for a child victim.[28] It remains to be seen how far the recommendations of the Pigot Committe, included in the 1991 Criminal Justice Act, have improved protection for child witnesses.

Further discouragement for victims to report offences comes from their treatment at the hands of the judiciary. Judges have doubted the extent of the victims' suffering: in sentencing a man for grabbing a woman by the throat in a pub forecourt and bolting her into a toilet before trying to rape her, Mr Justice Bristow, a judge at Birmingham Crown Court, commented that the experience had probably scarred the man more than it did his victim. Judges' comments in summing-up and sentencing have also been extremely critical of the conduct of victims or of their life-style, and have implied that by their dress, behaviour or their failure to resist they brought the offences on themselves. In 1988 at Lincoln Crown Court, Mr Justice Owen commented, while sentencing a 19-year-old man for raping a 12-year-old girl, that the girl had been 'asking for trouble' in going alone to his room.[29]

Finally, many victims fear the threat of the publicity that attends sexual trials. The Heilbron Advisory Group, set up by the Home Secretary in 1975, concluded that 'disclosure of a rape victim's name caused her great distress and also tended to discourage women from reporting alleged rape'.[30] The resulting Sexual Offences (Amendment) Act 1976 promised anonymity to the victims of rape (and to the defendant in a rape trial). However, this restriction does not apply to victims of other sexual offences, such as sexual assault or male rape. In these cases, a Press Council administered code of practice is meant to be complied with by newspapers.

In their analysis of the reporting of sexual crimes,[31] Keith Soothill and Sylvia Walby found that the anonymity restrictions established by the 1976 Act have had some impact. Newspapers tend to keep strictly to the letter of the law. However, in some cases, while the name of the victim is not reported, sufficient detail is given to enable victims to be identified, particularly where they come from small communities. Since the reporting restrictions do not apply to civil cases, victims can be – and are – identified there too. Finally, victims of non-rape cases can be named (unless they are juveniles), although Soothill and Walby's analysis reveals that the informal code of practice appears to be working well: out of the ninety-eight cases reported, only four victims were named.

However, as Soothill and Walby found, the media coverage of sex trials, like the comments of some judges, exhibits a tendency to place the responsibility for the offence upon the victim rather than the offender. Given the tradition of newspapers using sex in order to sell newspapers, and given the gender, background and experience of the legal establishment, a lack of sympathy and under- standing of the needs of victims who are predominantly female and young is hardly surprising. Nor is it surprising that they share the myths about the nature of sexual crime, myths which are themselves rein- forced through newspapers and judicial comments. However, the experience of victims in court and with the press is both distressing and destructive.

These fears – of arousing the antagonism of the perpetrator, family or the community, of meeting with an unsympathetic or disbelieving reception from the police, of being forced to relive the experience of the offence in minute and repeated detail during the trial, and of being depicted by defence barrister, judge and press as somehow responsible for the offence – all serve to discourage victims of sexual offences from reporting the offence. Indeed, what is possibly more surprising is that many victims do contact the police and pursue the case to the end.

Nevertheless, the reforms of police and court procedures, and the greater access for victims of assault to helplines and support systems, appear to have had a major impact on the reporting rate for sexual crime. The British Crime Survey estimates that, whereas at the time of the first survey in 1983 only 8.3 per cent of sexual assaults were being reported, by 1988 that figure had increased to 20.7 per cent. This increase in reporting rate alone would account for most of the increase in the official level of sexual crime over that period.[32]

POLICING PRACTICES

Although the reporting rate may be the major influence on the official level of sexual crime, the statistics can also be strongly influenced by the policies of the police. Some police practices serve to reduce the level of crime. Studies have shown that a disturbingly high proportion of rape reports are rejected by the police as having no basis in fact. An analysis of reports of rape received by Scotland Yard in 1990 revealed that 38 per cent of rape reports are listed as 'no crime'. In 28 per cent of cases so listed, the report was admitted to be false or withdrawn, and in 13 per cent the victim refused, was unwilling, or failed to substantiate the allegation. However, in 25 per cent of these cases the police decided that there was insufficient evidence, and in another 13 per cent the police believed that they had evidence that the allegation was false.[33] The belief that many reports of sexual crime are false and mendacious – a belief sustained by the press tendency to report a disproportionately large percentage of cases where apparent victims have lied[34] – appears deeply ingrained in the police.

Other police policies can inflate the figures. The quarterly figures issued by the Metropolitan Police on 13 September 1990 appeared to show a 5 per cent rise in the level of sexual offending in London in the third quarter of 1990. However, a closer analysis of the figures revealed that the increase was almost entirely the result of a police surveillance operation on a single public toilet in Slough. This operation resulted in some 300 offences being detected, all of which apparently involved consensual homosexual sex. These figures none the less caused London's *Evening Standard* to trumpet the headline: 'Sex, violent crimes soar.'[35]

Despite the fact that they can have a major impact on the official crime statistics, and through them, the public perception of sexual crime, no directions are given to the police by the Home Office about operations of this nature. In reply to a Parliamentary question in October 1991, Home Office Minister Peter Lloyd argued that: 'The priority and level of resources given to different kinds of investigation are operational matters for chief officers.'[36]

The policing policies towards sexual offending therefore vary from constabulary to constabulary, and from year to year, according to the culture and attitudes of individual police forces. Thus, policing of kerb-crawling differs greatly from county to county. Some forces – such as Cleveland and West Yorkshire – issue verbal warnings and ad hoc letters to kerb-crawlers. Others pursue aggressive prosecution policies; in 1989, Greater Manchester Police prosecuted 166 men for the offence.[37]

Changes in the cultures of individual police forces can have a direct impact on the crime statistics. In November 1991, the Metropolitan Police removed its bar on homosexuals joining the police force,[38] a move prompted by the formation of the Lesbian and Gay Police Association in June 1990 and by successful co-operation with the Lesbian and Gay Policing Initiative over the issue of 'queer-bashing'. This change in attitude was reflected in the 16 per cent reduction in the number of males arrested for gross indecency in London between July 1990 and July 1991. However, there is little room for complacency. There is some evidence to indicate that some police officers are deliberately disguising the extent of their operations against homosexual males by the use of obscure common-law statutes and by-laws. According to one newspaper article, two London men were recently charged under the 1860 Ecclesiastical Courts Jurisdiction Act with 'indecent behaviour in a churchyard'. They were acquitted when the local priest testified that the site of the arrest, a basement stairwell next to St Monica's Boxing Club, Hoxton, was not consecrated ground.[39]

Nor is there always any explicit policy to guide individual police officers in making decisions about whether or not to refer individual offenders for prosecution. Replying to a letter from Dawn Primarolo MP in December 1990, the Solicitor General Sir Nicholas Lyell MP confirmed that, in cases of homosexual sex, the decision was entirely at the discretion of the officer concerned. New Scotland Yard confirmed that no guidelines were issued to police officers on the subject: it was 'entirely up to the individual officer's discretion'.[40]

The priority given by some police forces to the policing of male homosexual behaviour and of prostitution is at odds with the concerns of the broader public. The public apparently considers that the police should give a high priority to combating sexual crime. In a survey conducted in 1990 as part of the Operational Police Review, sexual crime topped the list of offences which the public wanted the police to tackle. However, the sexual crimes concerned were violent assaults against women, not consensual homosexual sex or prostitution. It is perhaps significant that, in the same survey, combating violent assaults against women was not as important as domestic burglary and robbery on the police's own list of priorities.[41]

It is not only the attitudes and policies of the police which can influence the official level of sexual crime. The policies adopted by such agencies as the NSPCC, social work departments, victim support organizations, rape crisis centres, hospitals, schools and residential homes have a direct impact on crime statistics. As the furore over sexual crime – and particularly child sexual abuse – grows and the publicity accorded to it increases, so is the likelihood increased that workers in these agencies will recognize and act on the occurrence of signs of child sexual abuse. Following the recommendations of the report of the Butler-Sloss inquiry into the Cleveland child abuse scandal, the police are now more likely to be involved when cases are identified. According to a recent study of social services and police practice, four-fifths of police forces and three-quarters of social services departments now work together investigating child sexual abuse allegations.[42]

It is uncertain what effect the routine involvement of the police in investigating allegations of child sexual abuse in Britain will have on the rate of reported crime. Practice in Germany and Holland, and to a lesser extent in France, Belgium and Sweden, shies away from the involvement of the police and the threat of prosecution. Supporters of this system argue that the involvement of the police and the threat of prosecution reduces the likelihood of offenders, or others concerned, reporting the occurrence of the abuse and coming forward for treatment. When the Kind in Nood clinic in Brussels decided to end their co-operation with the police, the number of self-referrals to the clinic jumped from 3 per cent to 30 per cent.[43]

However, even in Europe this approach has not always been met with full agreement from the authorities: one therapist in Antwerp has been prosecuted for failing to report a case of child abuse to the police. It is a policy which meets with little support and sympathy from supporters of the feminist analysis of sexual offending. They argue that sexual abuse is a crime like any other, and criminal investigation and prosecution are necessary to demonstrate both to the victim and to society that abuse is not to be tolerated.

NON-OFFICIAL STATISTICS: VICTIM SURVEYS AND RANDOM SAMPLES

The disincentives for victims to report abuse, police practices and the policies of other authorities all make the official statistics a very inaccurate guide to the real level of sexual crime. Set against these distorted figures is the picture indicated by victim surveys. This picture is very different to the one shown in the official statistics.

Surveys which attempt to reveal the hidden figure of sexual crime have their own particular problems. Many of them are surveys conducted in the USA, which may not be applicable to Britain. The methodology of many of these surveys is questionable, and few use representative (statistically random) samples. The definitions they use of what is, and is not, sexual crime are often not given in sufficient detail, and few employ definitions that can be compared with other surveys. The surveys also require that respondents are prepared to reveal fully and honestly the number and nature of the crimes of which they have been a victim. The number of offences revealed often crucially depends upon the victim defining them as crimes: there may be little agreement about what constitutes full 'consent' or what constitutes a sexual assault. Finally, few are repeated surveys, so it is almost impossible to draw conclusions across time to discover whether sexual offending is increasing or decreasing.

The largest-scale British surveys of the extent of crime are the British Crime Surveys. These are based upon interviews with 11,000 (statistically random) members of the general public, with interviewers asking a standard set of questions. According to the British Crime Survey, the number of sexual offences committed is far higher than the official statistics indicate: the BCS figures show 60,000 sexual offences being committed in 1987, compared with an official figure of 25,000. However, far from showing an increase in the level of sexual crime, the BCS shows sexual crime declining between the time of the first survey in 1983 and that conducted in 1987. As has been said, the authors explain the discrepancy largely by an increase in reporting.[44] However, it is possible that police and other policies have also had an impact.

The conclusions of the British Crime Survey have been severely questioned. The interviews from which the findings were derived took place in the interviewees' own homes and were in many cases conducted by male interviewers. This may have discouraged disclosure of such personal and private experiences. Certainly the level of sexual offending revealed by the surveys has been very low – no rapes and only one attempted rape in the 1983 survey. Other surveys have shown widely differing rates of sexual assaults. One American survey of assaults on adults found that around 45 per cent of Californian women had been the victim of a rape or attempted rape.[45] In Britain, a 1982 survey by Women Against Rape found that of 1,236 women who responded to a questionnaire (2,000 had been originally given a questionnaire – a response rate of 62 per cent), no less than 214 (17 per cent) said that they had been raped, and 243 (20 per cent) that they had been the victims of an attempted rape. In only 8 per cent of the cases had the incident been reported to the police.[46] On the other hand, in a survey conducted by *Company* magazine, only 10 per cent of respondents reported that they had been the victim of sexual assault, rape or attempted rape. Here, the reporting rate was only 3 per cent.[47]

These surveys were all aimed primarily at adult women, and given that the methodology employed in the British surveys involved asking women to fill in and return a questionnaire, their results may be even less than usually reliable. No comparable surveys have been carried out to investigate the level of offending against adult males. However, some indications can be gleaned from the fact that one local support group, London Survivors, deals with over 1,000 new cases each year.[48] Martin Dockrell of London Survivors estimates that there are around 6,000 cases a year in London alone, only one-tenth of which are reported to the police.[49]

Surveys seeking to assess the rate of child sexual abuse have produced a similarly wide range of offending rates. Once again, the majority are from the USA, peaking with Wyatt's finding that 62 per cent of girls had been victims.[50] Other surveys found that only 7 per cent of children had been abused.[51] In Britain, Baker and Duncan revealed a victimization rate of 10 per cent, but their methodology has been much criticized.[52] A BBC Childwatch survey found rates as low as 3 per cent. On the other hand, two studies by Nash and West revealed rates for girls of between 42 and 54 per cent.[53] Finally, the extensive survey for the Child Abuse Studies Unit by Kelly, Regan and Burton, whose final results have yet to be published, found that 59 per cent of females and 27 per cent of males reported at least one unwanted sexual experience before the age of 18. Using a more restrictive definition of abuse (to exclude such offences as 'flashing'), the rates were 21 per cent and 7 per cent respectively.[54]

The disparities between the extent of sexual offending claimed in these studies provides little confidence in their accuracy. In part, this may reflect the fact that few of their samples were truly random. However, even if one were to take a conservative view and rule out the higher estimates of victimization, it still appears to be the case that at least one-quarter of women and perhaps one in ten men have been victims of sexual assaults. Few of those offences will be reported to the authorities and fewer still of the reports will find their way into the official crime statistics.

These surveys also reveal that the reality of rape and sexual abuse is different from the popular image, and that the sorts of cases which result in conviction are exceptional in nature. In a study of the patterns of rape, Lorna Smith of the Home Office Research and Planning Unit[55] found that two-fifths of the rapes were carried out by individuals known to the victims (e.g. former or current husbands or boyfriends, or friends); in only 32 per cent of cases was the rapist a total stranger. This echoes a finding from the London Rape Crisis Centre that as many as two-thirds of victims know their rapist.[56] Nor did the location of the rapes accord with the popular stereotype. The majority of the rapes examined by Smith took place indoors, in the victim's or offender's home, or in another house known to the victim. Only 18 per cent took place in public locations.

The findings of studies such as Smith's are unambiguous. Rape is not usually a product of the street, and the principal threat is not from strangers. Victims are most at risk from people they know, in environments they know. The cases which reach court and result in conviction are very different. In Grubin and Gunn's study of imprisoned rapists, less than half of the sample knew their victims, and in only 7 per cent of cases had there been an intimate relationship between the two. Less than a quarter of the rapes had taken place after some social contact between rapist and offender; in over half the cases, the victim had been attacked in the street or the offender had broken into her home.[57]

It is the same with child abuse. Both the popular image and the pattern which emerges from official statistics is that the threat posed to children comes principally from adult strangers, and, to a far lesser extent, from incest. However, the Child Abuse Studies Unit report found that only 14 per cent of child victims were abused by strangers. The majority of the abusers were relatives or people known to the victims. None of the major general population studies of child abuse shows high levels of incestuous abuse, and the Child Abuse Studies Unit report found only 24 cases (2 per cent).[58] There is also increasing evidence to indicate that many of the abusers of children are young people. The Child Abuse Studies Unit found that 27 per cent of the abuse they uncovered was committed by adolescents aged between 13 and 17. Two surveys analysed by a committee set up by the National Children's Home both found that over 35 per cent of cases of child abuse were committed by people under the age of 19.[59]

The disparity between the picture revealed by surveys and the types of cases which come before the courts and result in convictions clearly reflects the nature of the types of offences which are likely to be reported to the authorities. As has been said, it may be difficult for victims to report cases where the abuser is someone known to them. However, the disparity also reflects the effect of police, prosecution and court processes.

PROSECUTIONS AND CAUTIONS

Once an offence is reported, there are still many stages before an offender is convicted and sentenced. The offender has to be identified and a decision taken about whether there is sufficient evidence to prosecute. In some cases, it may be decided that prosecution is not in the public interest and the offender may be cautioned, or diverted from the criminal justice system altogether. Finally, when the case comes to court, the offender may be acquitted.

The attrition rate for sexual offences reported to the police and those which result in convictions is extraordinarily high. As a result, few offenders who commit sexual crimes are ever convicted in court. A striking example of this process was recorded by David Wright: Wright studied 255 rapes and attempted rapes investigated by the police, involving 240 men. A total of 204 men were actually arrested, of whom 201 eventually appeared before the courts. Twenty-two were found guilty of rape and thirteen of attempted rape. Another sixty-five were convicted of other offences connected with the rapes or attempted rapes, mostly of lesser offences.[60]

The pattern identified by Wright is borne out in official statistics. The 3,305 cases of rape recorded by the police in 1989 in

England and Wales resulted in only 613 offenders being
cautioned or convicted; 15,376 recorded indecent assaults on
females produced 4,119 convicted or cautioned offenders. In all,
22,215 recorded sexual offences resulted in 10,729 offenders being
cautioned or convicted.[61] Unless many of these offenders are
being convicted of multiple sexual crimes, it is clear that only a
small proportion of recorded sexual offences result in the
offender being brought to justice.

Much of the gap between the number of criminal offences
recorded and the number of offenders convicted can of course
usually be explained by the failure of the police to identify the
criminals. For most offences, police clear-up rates are disturbingly
low – 31 per cent of thefts, 26 per cent of burglaries, 23 per cent of
cases of criminal damage. However, this is not true of sexual offending. Many offenders are known to their victims, and many sexual
crimes are detected because of direct police action. Only a relatively
small percentage of sexual offences therefore are not cleared up: in
the past ten years, the clear-up rate has never dropped below 70 per
cent. A similar pattern can be seen in crimes of non-sexual violence,
where the attacker is often already known to the victim.

However, the fact that the police know – or believe that they
know – the identity of the offender does not automatically
guarantee that prosecution will follow. The failure to prosecute
will usually be for two reasons: either the evidence may be insufficient to guarantee a conviction, or it may be thought against
the public interest to prosecute. In the latter case, there is the
option to institute an official caution.

Since 1986, decisions about prosecution for sexual offences
have been the responsibility of the Crown Prosecution Service;
until that time, the decision was entirely in the hands of the
police, with the exception of cases of incest or consensual
buggery between two males, one of whom was under the age of
21, where the Director of Public Prosecutions was responsible.
Considerable variation in police policy as regard to cautioning
and prosecution resulted, and it has been suggested that the
result of this variation reduced the number of sexual offences
prosecuted. A more consistent approach would have resulted in
more sexual offenders coming before the courts.[62]

Cautioning and non-prosecution on public interest grounds are
dealt with in the CPS *Code for Crown Prosecutors*. Prosecutors are
advised to consider the ages of the participants, their ages relative

to each other, and whether or not there was 'any element of seduction or corruption' in the commission of the offence. Sexual assaults on children and offences against adults such as rape 'which amount to gross personal violation' should almost always result in prosecution as long as sufficient evidence is available.[63]

The change from police prosecution to prosecution by the CPS has not had a noticeable effect on the number of offenders who are cautioned rather than prosecuted: there has been a slow growth in the number of offenders cautioned for sexual offences since 1979, but this is against a background of an equal growth in the number of offences being recorded. In 1989, some 3,500 individuals received a caution for a sexual offence, around one-third of all those convicted or cautioned for sexual offending. It is clear that the guideline relating to the age of the offender is being closely observed. In 1989, 92 per cent of boys aged between 10 and 14, and 78 per cent of boys between 14 and 17 convicted or cautioned for a sexual offence were cautioned rather than prosecuted.

These figures show a surprisingly high level of diversion from prosecution. Nevertheless, there has been some pressure for the policy of discontinuance of prosecution on public interest grounds to be widened. In particular, it has been argued that the policy of initiating prosecution in all cases of child sexual abuse is counter-productive. Lord Justice Butler-Sloss recognized the possibility that the knowledge that they faced prosecution might deter some offenders from coming forward voluntarily:

> Some consideration might be given in certain circumstances to the wider interests of the child and family and whether different arrangements might be made in suitable cases for those abusers who admit their guilt, who co-operate with the arrangements for the child and who are prepared to submit themselves to a programme of control.[64]

This is the policy in many other European jurisdictions. In Holland, prosecution is waived on condition that the offender attend 20–25 two-hour therapy sessions over a seven-month period. No such schemes exist in Britain, and an attempt by the private Gracewell Clinic in Birmingham to offer treatment to unconvicted offenders has been hampered by disagreements about who would pay their fees.[65]

In many cases, prosecution will be dropped on evidential grounds. In only a few cases of sexual abuse are there physical signs that abuse has taken place; and even where signs are evident, they are rarely conclusive.[66] In practice, it is often the word of the victim against that of the abuser, and where the offender steadfastly denies the offence, or where the accuser is a child and the accused an adult, or where there has been a prior relationship and the question is one of consent, that may not be enough. It is not possible simply to assume that the gap between the number of offences recorded and the number of offenders prosecuted or cautioned represents the number of offences not proceeded with on the grounds of evidence. Many of them may form the basis of multiple prosecutions or offences 'taken into consideration'. However, it is likely that in many of these cases the CPS has decided that there is insufficient evidence to proceed. In many of the cases of child abuse, the only option may be to remove the child from the home, thereby punishing the abused rather than the abuser.

CONVICTION OR ACQUITTAL?

Even where cases are brought to court, many do not result in a conviction. A high proportion of offenders who are prosecuted willingly plead guilty: one (now rather old) survey found that nine out of ten of those accused of incest pleaded guilty.[67] However, this is by no means true of all offenders. In particular, most individuals accused of rape plead not guilty in court, and with considerable success: less than half of rape prosecutions are successful in gaining a conviction. Indeed, the likelihood of being convicted of an offence of rape has been declining steeply over the past few years: the proportion of men acquitted or not proceeded against following a first appearance at a Magistrates' Court has risen from 38 per cent in 1980 to 58 per cent in 1988. A similar proportion of child abuse cases are unsuccessful.[68]

These statistics are a considerable cause for concern, but are hardly surprising in view of the factors discussed above. Court practices and the sheer difficulty of proving the lack of consent have bedevilled attempts to make rape accusations be upheld in court. Child abuse cases have been hampered by the difficulty of finding ways in which children's testimony can be elicited without bias and used in court to support an accusation, while still allowing the defendant the right to question what is being said. Despite the increased willingness to tailor court proceedings to the needs of child witnesses, such as the use of screens to protect the child from sight of the defendant, child abuse cases still fall when the child's testimony is exposed to the rigours of cross-examination.[69]

The difficulty in obtaining convictions in child abuse cases which depended upon the evidence of the children themselves prompted the setting up of the Pigot Inquiry in 1989, many of whose recommendations were included in the 1991 Criminal Justice Act. Children's evidence can now be given via video links, and recorded testimony from children can now be accepted in limited circumstances, thus rendering cross-examination by the defence impossible. In addition, in order to spare victims of sexual crime (both adults and children) the necessity of undergoing the ordeal of testifying on two occasions, the right of defendants in sexual trials to test the evidence against them in full committal hearings in the Magistrates' Court can now be overridden in the interest of the witnesses.

The measures in the Criminal Justice Act were finally implemented in October 1992, and it is too early to judge how effective they have proved. However, the changes may also have unfortunate consequences. The removal of such safeguards as the right to a full hearing before committal to Crown Court – enjoyed by individuals accused of any other sort of offence – places defendants in sex trials in a uniquely disadvantaged position. Defendants' inability to have the evidence against them fully tested in court before their eventual trial date may well condemn them to longer periods on remand in custody than they would have otherwise had to suffer. However, as was made clear during the passage of the Bill, there are few votes in preserving the legal safeguards of those accused of sexual offences at the expense of victims. Despite the risk of miscarriages of justice, it is clear that the need to address the concerns of vulnerable witnesses has taken priority.

In any event, the new protections for witnesses may do little to change the fact that the criminal justice process gives a victim of sexual crime little hope of seeing the abuser brought to justice. Given the unlikelihood of any rape or sexual assault they commit ever being reported to the police, given the reluctance of some police officers to believe the report and to record the crime, given the possibility of their identity not being discovered or of there being insufficient evidence to prosecute, and given the marked reluctance of juries to convict for many sexual crimes, sexual offenders who end up convicted of their crimes are unusual cases indeed. Such a travesty of justice is scant consolation for a victim.

Chapter 3

Sentencing: just deserts and public protection

The increase in the number of sexual offences being reported and recorded has created what, in other areas, the criminologist Professor Stanley Cohen has labelled a 'moral panic' about sexual offending. Media reporting has given the impression that there has been an unprecedented explosion in sexual crime, and that women and children are increasingly at risk of attack by sexual monsters. This has been supported by politicians anxious to play the law and order card, and their call for tougher treatment for sex offenders has gone largely unopposed. The result has been significant hardening of sentencing policy towards sexual offenders.

Such panics about crime often have a direct impact upon the penalties applied to offenders by the courts. In *Hooligan: A History of Respectable Fears*,[1] Geoffrey Pearson traced the creation of successive panics about the apparent threat posed by criminal youths and the impact upon the penal policy of the age. For example, the introduction of flogging in the 'Garrotters Act' of 1863 was a direct response to media reports of a spate of street robberies. Perhaps more significantly, the panic was followed by a wider retreat from the notion of rehabilitation, with the introduction of minimum sentences of five years for second-time offenders. The parallels with 1992's rushed legislation introducing tougher penalties to counter media-generated fears of 'joy-riding' are obvious.

PANIC AND MEDIA REPORTING

The media panic about sexual crime has been deeper and more sustained than the recent short-lived obsessions with contemporary youth cults such as joy-riding and warehouse 'raves'.

Since the beginnings of a popular press, sexual crime has always proved a fruitful source of stories. However, as Soothill and Walby have demonstrated,[2] there has been a steady increase in the number of sexual crimes reported in the media over the past few years, with the most significant increase coming between the years 1971 and 1978. Moreover, whereas in 1951 stories about rape were almost all confined to one newspaper, the *News of the World*, by 1985 even the broadsheets were feeding their readers on a regular diet of rape stories. Indeed, page 3 of the *Daily Telegraph* now rivals page 3 of the *Sun* for its obsession with sex.

The nature of the reporting of sexual crime has also changed. In the 1950s and 1960s, few details of any sexual crime were reported. Euphemisms were used – rape was referred to as 'carnal knowledge'. In recent years, however, newspapers have begun to go into considerable detail and to use reports of sexual crime as part of a semi-pornographic 'package'. One common strategy has been to place reports of sex crimes next to pictures of topless women. In one case, the *Sunday Sport* featured on its front page a story purporting to tell of a model's multiple rape, and followed it with an invitation for readers to ring a pay-line number where more explicit details would be given.

The effect of these changes has been to move sexual crime from the realms of the extraordinary into the everyday. Stories about rape and child abuse are now the staples of newspaper reportage: in 1985, according to Soothill and Walby, papers like the *Sun* were averaging one rape story a week, and there is no reason to believe that this average has declined. These accounts also build up the image of perpetrators of sexual crime as modern-day monsters. Offenders such as Malcolm Fairley, who raped and assaulted men and women during a series of burglaries in the early 1980s, are given nicknames (in Fairley's case 'The Fox') and become fully developed folk devils capable of any vice. Offenders who commit assaults on children receive similar treatment. The equation of sexual offender and monster is now firmly part of the public psyche. 'Monster' and 'beast' are common euphemisms for sex offenders in the prison system.

To a certain extent, this tendency towards portraying sexual offenders as monsters has been encouraged by many of those working with them. Those working with sex offenders (as with other types of offender) inevitably gain a deeper understanding of the extent and seriousness of their prior offending, and of their potential dangerousness. The current analytical model of sex offenders' behaviour – the myths about women and children, the planning, the grooming of potential victims, the denial – lends itself to a view of sex offenders as somehow more cold-blooded, more conniving, more manipulative than other offenders. It is also a powerful strategy in the quest for funding and support for work with individuals who are so hated to emphasize the danger that many of them present to the public.

The reporting of sexual crime has a direct impact on the level of public fear. Fear of sexual crime seems to be increasing: the number of women reporting to the British Crime Survey that they were very fearful of being the victim of a sexual attack increased from 23 per cent in 1982 to 30 per cent in 1984.[3] However, one should not push this finding too far: there is some evidence that the public increasingly perceives itself as being at risk of becoming a victim of crime of all sorts. Nevertheless, there are indications that the fear of sexual crime has largely been driven by media coverage, rather than by personal experience.[4]

The increasing public fear of crime has been blamed in part on the issuing of the crime statistics on a quarterly basis, giving the impression of an inexorable rise in crime. In 1991 a working party of newspaper editors, police, and Home Office officials recommended wholesale changes in the way in which crime statistics are published.[5] However, changes in reporting practices will come about only slowly, and will be faced with considerable opposition from within the media themselves. On 13 September 1990 the quarterly crime statistics were issued with the caveat that the British Crime Survey had suggested that the official figures misrepresented the true changes in crime levels. Most newspapers chose to ignore the caveat and headline the rise in the figures on violent and sexual crime. The refusal to countenance a change in the way in which the quarterly crime figures were reported has also contributed to the departure of the Home Affairs Correspondent from one national broadsheet newspaper. It is not only official reports on the level of sexual crime which are misused. Figures given in the 1985 NSPCC report *Trends in Child Abuse* were inflated by many newspapers, and many of them linked the report to the murder of a young girl, Leone Keating, to emphasize the threat posed to children by strangers. Similarly, much of the reporting of the WAR survey *Ask Any Woman* chose to focus on the issue of whether women should carry weapons for self-protection. The effect of such reporting was subtly to increase the level of public fear of sexual crime, and to perpetuate the belief that the principal threat to women and children is posed by strangers.

'CASTRATE THE BUGGERS'

The belief that the public is increasingly at risk from sexual offences and the labelling of many who perpetrate them as 'monsters' and 'fiends' has fuelled calls for changes in the sentencing of sexual offenders. Newspapers have been loud in their demands for tougher treatment for sexual offenders. In 1985, the *Daily Mail* commented in its editorial:

> Rape is a growing problem in Britain. What is needed . . . is swingeing penalties. There should be exemplary punishments to stamp on the present horrifying trend towards associating burglary with rape. There should also be severe minimum sentences to ensure that no guilty party gets off lightly. Rape is a particularly beastly crime and the law should fully mirror public revulsion.[6]

These have been backed with clarion calls from MPs such as Geoffrey Dickens, who, in a speech to the Conservative Party Conference in October 1991, demanded:

> If you want to stop child abuse and rape of women, pass legislation and, on the second offence – not the first in case there is a mistake – put it before Parliament that you can castrate the buggers.

As the rapturous reception given to Geoffrey Dickens' speech indicates, these efforts have built a powerful lobby for a 'get tough' policy. This feeds into and is supported by more general demands for tougher sentencing of crime in general. The image of sex offenders walking free from courts is used by newspapers as part of a more general campaign for a harder line towards offenders: in 1992 the *Evening Standard* reported then Home Secretary Kenneth Baker's electioneering call for restrictions on bail for car offenders and burglars with the call 'Don't Free Men on Rape Charge'.[7]

In one recent case, the police have also become involved in promoting tougher sentencing for sexual crime. In February 1993, a 15-year-old boy was sentenced at Newport Crown Court to three years' supervision and ordered to pay £500 compensation to the victim 'to give her a good holiday'. The chief constable of Gwent, John Over, called the sentence 'woefully inadequate' and sought a meeting with the Crown Prosecution Service to arrange for an appeal against the leniency of the sentence.[8] The appeal was duly heard and the sentence was increased to two years' detention in a Young Offenders' Institution.

It is noticeable, however, that these calls for tougher sentencing have been met with only limited support from groups representing the victims of sexual offences. Caroline Coleman argued in a letter to the *Guardian* that it was entirely wrong to classify groups like Women Against Rape in the same bracket as 'rent-a-quote politicians' calling for longer sentences:

> In the past week, as often before, we have spent hours patiently explaining to incredulous journalists that rape neither begins nor ends with sentencing. For ten years WAR has been under heavy pressure from the law-and-order lobby to make rape a lever for higher sentences (for all crimes), hanging, castration, sexual repression, state censorship and worse. We have never obliged . . .[9]

Nevertheless, not only has the call for tougher sentencing gone largely unresisted by those groups who are usually loud in their opposition to such moves, but it has received the active support of many of those working with sex offenders. The National Association of Probation Officers, an organization with a proud tradition of opposing moves to increase sentence lengths, voted down a motion at their 1991 Annual Conference which had proposed diversion from custody for minor sexual offenders. Two rationales for supporting longer sentences for sex offenders were advanced during that debate. On the one hand, delegates expressed the view that, in the past, sexual offences had been undervalued in comparison with other – especially property – offences: custodial sentences had been more frequent, and longer, for offences of robbery and burglary than for rape and sexual assault. On the other, it was argued that all sex offenders are potentially dangerous individuals, and that the imposition of long custodial sentences would at least have the effect of removing them from society for a period of time.

Both of these arguments have a degree of force. It is certainly true that, in the past, the courts have often treated sexual offences as significantly less serious than offences against property. In 1980, 58 per cent of adult males convicted of sex offences at Crown Court were sentenced to immediate custody; the average sentence length was 30.2 months. In the same year, 64 per cent of those convicted of burglary and 87 per cent of those convicted of robbery were imprisoned; the average sentence lengths were 17.4 months for burglary and 38.5 for robbery.[10] Sometimes this can be taken to absurd lengths: the judge who sentenced two defendants in the 1985 Ealing vicarage rape case to three and five years (describing the trauma suffered by the victim as 'not so very great') passed a three-year sentence on a pickpocket shortly afterwards.

The distress that such relative undervaluing of their suffering causes to survivors of sexual assault is deep and abiding. However, the undervaluing of the seriousness of sexual offences relative to property offences does not automatically demand that sentence lengths for sexual offenders should be increased. There are grounds for arguing that, rather than increasing the severity of sentences for sex offenders, sentences handed out to those who have committed property offences should be reduced. It has long been argued by penal reform groups that too many property offenders are imprisoned, and for too long. To a degree, these arguments have been acknowledged by Government: the original intention of the 1991 Criminal Justice Act was to divert more property offenders from the prison system, and the Act itself contained measures such as the lowering of maximum penalties for some property offences. If that intention had been adhered to, the relativity could have been reversed without a marked increase in sentence lengths for sex offenders.

The second argument, that all sex offenders are potentially dangerous and that longer sentences would disable them by removing them from society, also must be taken seriously. Many sex offenders who come before the courts have been offending for many years and undoubtedly pose a continuing risk to society. The argument that they must be locked away from society has been advanced with some force by many of those working with sex offenders. Such a policy, it is argued, will also provide the advocates of treatment with sufficient time to tackle offenders' behaviour. Writing in *Behavioural Sciences and the Law*, Bill Marshall, Director of the Kingston Sexual Behaviour Clinic in Canada, and a man who acted as a consultant to the Prison Service in setting up the sex offender treatment programme in British prisons, argued that:

Many sex offenders constitute such a serious threat to innocent women and children, that they must be held in a secure setting to protect society, at least while they are being treated . . . We should certainly sentence more of these men to jail and give them all a sentence which is commensurate with their crime, not only to provide some satisfaction to the victims and society, but also to allow for a sufficient length of incarceration to permit adequate treatment to occur.[11]

This argument is not without its problems. A doctrine of the sort Marshall is advocating does not easily sit with our notions of justice. The nature of the offender's punishment, he is arguing, should not simply be determined by the seriousness of the offence, but by the risk the offender poses to society and the length of time that will be needed in prison to provide adequate treatment. Offenders will be imprisoned not because of what they have done – they may have committed only minor sexual crimes – but on the basis of what they might do at some future date, or for a length of time to be determined by the therapist. That is at odds with the notion, fundamental to the concept of justice, that there should be some degree of proportionality between the crime and the punishment, and that the length of sentence should be determined by the judiciary.

JUDICIAL POLICY AND JUDICIAL PRACTICE

The effect of this pressure upon the judicial policy towards the sentencing of sex offenders appears clear. The repeated criticisms of the inconsistent and insulting sentences handed out by some judges led to the then Lord Chief Justice, Lord Lane, issuing a guideline judgement in the case of *R. v Roberts* in January 1982 (only a few days after one judge, Judge Richards at Ipswich Crown Court, had sentenced a rapist to a fine). In this judgement, Lord Lane set out the guideline sentences he expected judges to use in sentencing rape offenders. Rape was always to be treated as a serious crime, and other than in 'wholly exceptional circumstances' it should be met with a custodial sentence. Sentence should be longer if there were aggravating features such as the use of a weapon, threats or additional violence, if the victim was elderly or very young, if there was a breach of trust or the offender had broken into the victim's home, if other sexual acts were performed, or if other people were involved.

Unfortunately, Lord Lane neglected to indicate what the appropriate sentence for each aggravated category should be. As a result, sentences for rape continued to vary wildly. A man who twice raped a 6-year-old girl was sentenced at Leeds Crown Court in 1985 to twelve months, with eight months of that suspended; released after 25 days, he met his victim in the street soon afterwards and she ran home in hysterics.[12] This initial guideline judgement had to be amplified further in 1986 in the case of *R. v Billam*, with five years being the starting-point for rape without any aggravating features, eight years for those who break in to rape, and fifteen years for multiple rapists.

In August 1989, while hearing one of the first of the appeals against sentence brought by the Attorney General, Lord Lane took the opportunity of issuing a similar guideline judgement to cover cases of incestuous child abuse. As with rape, the length of sentence to be passed varied according to the circumstances of the case: the age of the child, the length of time the abuse had been taking place, whether threats had been used, and so on. For example, the starting-point for any sentence for the incestuous abuse of a girl under 13 would be six years' imprisonment.

The impact on the actual sentencing policy adopted by magistrates and judges appears just as marked. Tables 3.1 to 3.4 list the sentences given for various sexual offences in 1980, 1985 and 1989. Taken from the official Home Office list of sexual offences, they nevertheless exclude offences relating to bigamy and prostitution. In order to reveal the differences in the patterns of sentencing, they are divided into four major groups: rape and sexual assaults; sex with minors; incest; and homosexual offences.

As can be seen, since 1980 there has been a marked increase in the percentage of sex offenders sentenced to custody by the courts: in 1980, 18 per cent of all sex offenders received immediate custodial sentences; by 1989, that had increased to 33 per cent (having hit a peak of 37 per cent in 1987). It is clear that, at least insofar as the use of custody is concerned, sentencers' policy markedly hardened during the 1980s.

The variations in the sentencing of the different classes of sexual crime must be treated with some caution. There is often considerable variation in prosecution practice as to precisely what charge is preferred against, say, a blood relative committing an assault on a child or a man having sex with a 16-year-old youth. Nevertheless, it is clear that the general pressure towards an increased use of

Table 3.1 Rape and sexual assault on adults, 1980–1989

Offence/Sentence	1980	1985	1989
(A) *Rape*			
Absolute/conditional discharge	–	–	1
Fine	–	–	1
Probation order/ supervision order	3	–	4
Community service	3	–	1
Suspended sentence	4	5	2
Imprisonment	302	319	445
Other	23	18	22
Total	335	342	476
(B) *Indecent assault (female)*			
Absolute/conditional discharge	314	258	244
Fine	644	292	323
Probation order/ supervision order	465	459	531
Community service	30	42	47
Suspended sentence	241	213	319
Imprisonment	416	661	1,004
Other	307	215	204
Total	2,444	2,140	2,672
(C) *Indecent assault (male)*			
Absolute/conditional discharge	130	95	139
Fine	326	178	254
Probation order/ supervision order	133	150	169
Community service	13	21	23
Suspended sentence	59	65	117
Imprisonment	114	197	337
Other	99	68	89
Total	874	774	1,118

Table 3.2 Sex with minors, 1980–1989

Offence/Sentence	1980	1985	1989
(A) *Unlawful sexual intercourse:*			
Girl under 16			
Absolute/conditional discharge	96	76	42
Fine	212	79	65
Probation order/			
supervision order	44	59	27
Community service	27	25	15
Suspended sentence	82	43	30
Imprisonment	86	103	86
Other	14	12	4
Total	561	397	262
(B) *Unlawful sexual intercourse:*			
Girl under 13			
Absolute/conditional discharge	5	5	5
Fine	8	2	3
Probation order/			
supervision order	16	9	7
Community service	–	12	1
Suspended sentence	14	10	9
Imprisonment	50	70	61
Other	9	2	8
Total	102	110	96
(C) *Gross indecency with children*			
Absolute/conditional discharge	23	17	13
Fine	54	29	23
Probation order/			
supervision order	79	95	70
Community service	–	3	7
Suspended sentence	52	32	25
Imprisonment	37	79	68
Other	20	14	13
Total	265	269	219

Table 3.3 Buggery and indecency (males), 1980–1989

	1980	1985	1989
Absolute/conditional discharge	138	110	170
Fine	1,380	561	1,240
Probation order/supervision order	54	44	55
Community service	3	9	5
Suspended sentence	81	37	46
Imprisonment	151	192	211
Other	33	20	29
Total	1,840	973	1,756

Table 3.4 Incest

	1980	1985	1989
Absolute/conditional discharge	3	–	3
Fine	2	–	3
Probation order/supervision order	3	1	1
Community service	1	1	1
Suspended sentence	20	21	6
Imprisonment	97	96	134
Other	5	2	6
Total	145	128	166

custody has had a more direct impact on particular classes of sexual crime than on others. Unsurprisingly, the percentage use of custody has increased has shown its greatest increase in those types of offence where previously there was a low use of custody. In cases of indecency with children, the incidence of custody has increased from 14 to 31 per cent; in cases of indecent assaults on females, the increase has been from 17 to 38 per cent. In the case of such offences as rape and incest, which in 1980 already had imprisonment rates of 90 and 67 per cent respectively, the increase has been less marked: to 94 per cent and 81 per cent.

The increase in the use of custody has been largely at the expense of the use of the fine. Whereas in 1980, 212 (38 per cent) of the 561 offenders sentenced for unlawful sexual intercourse with a girl under 16 (USI) were fined, by 1989 the proportion fined had fallen to 25 per cent. Such a drop could, of course, be the natural result of the decline in the number of offenders being prosecuted for USI: an increased use of the prosecution's power not to initiate proceedings against less serious cases would have an immediate impact on the use of the less punitive disposals. However, the decline in the use of the fine also shows itself in other offences. The proportion of offenders convicted of (non-rape) adult sexual assaults who received fines fell from 29.2 per cent in 1980 to 15.2 per cent in 1989. In part, this may reflect a general decline in the use of the fine to punish crime: whereas in 1980, 48 per cent of all offenders were fined, by 1989 that had fallen to 40 per cent. However, the fall in the number of fines for sexual offences far exceeds the general fall and may reflect a more punitive attitude on the part of the courts.

The figures also point up the failure of the probation service to intervene to any significant extent in diverting sexual offenders from custody. The proportion of sexual offenders placed on probation has shown little increase over the decade: in 1980, 11 per cent of offenders received probation orders; by 1989 the figure had risen to 12 per cent (although in the intervening years it had been higher). The role of the probation service in intervening with sexual offenders forms the subject of a later chapter; nevertheless, it is worth noting here that the ambivalence, reflected at the NAPO debate discussed earlier, about whether sexual offenders should be diverted from custody at all may have had an impact on probation officers' willingness to argue forcefully for probation supervision.

The general pattern of harsher sentencing of sexual offenders is also reflected in the average length of the custodial sentences passed by the courts (Table 3.5).

As can be seen from Table 3.5, there has been a general and sustained increase in sentence lengths for sexual offences. Average sentence lengths increased from 44 to 75 months for rape, from 35 to 43 months for incest, and from 12 to 22 months for indecent assault. The increases were particularly marked in the more serious offences, those which were sentenced at Crown Courts. Sentence lengths at Magistrates' Courts on the other hand remained relatively stable.

Table 3.5 Average length (months) of sentence of immediate imprisonment, 1980–1988*

	1980	1985	1989
Rape	44	54	75
Indecent assaults (females)	12	14	21
Indecent assaults (males)	8.5	11	20
USI (girl under 16)	10	10	21
USI (girl under 13)	31	25	38
Gross indecency (children)	10.5	11	10
Buggery/indecency (males)	33	32	42
Incest	35	30	43

* These do not include life sentences of which there were: in 1980, 4 for rape and 2 for buggery/indecency; in 1985, 9 for rape and 1 for indecent assault; in 1989, 12 for rape, 6 for buggery/ indecency and 1 for indecent assault.

Nevertheless, there are two slight exceptions to this general pattern of harsher sentencing. The sentencing of homosexual offences, particularly buggery and indecency between males, which cover the majority of offences involving consensual homosexual sex, has not shown the same proportionate rise in the use of custody. Although there has been an increase in the average length of sentence for buggery and indecency between males, the proportion of prison sentences has scarcely increased. In 1980, 8 per cent of those convicted of these offences were sentenced to custody; by 1989, the proportion had only risen by 4 per cent. It appears on a superficial reading of the statistics that the furore over sexual offending appears to have had little impact upon the sentencing of people convicted of consensual homosexual sex.

Despite this, the sentencing of consensual homosexual sex is a matter for considerable concern. A detailed analysis (by Peter Tatchell from the campaigning homosexual group Outrage) of the sentencing of offences of buggery, soliciting and indecency has shown that during 1989 approximately 90-100 men were imprisoned for consensual homosexual sex with men over the age of 16. During the period 1980–89, 2,156 males (including 178 males aged between 13 and 21) were imprisoned for consenting homosexual sex. The sentences passed on these men were up to twice as long as those passed on men having consensual sex with girls aged between 13 and 16.[13] This represented a marked increase in the length of custodial sentencing. The average length of sentence for buggery and indecency was static in the Magistrates' Courts, but rose from 34 to 42 months in the Crown Courts. However, the offence of buggery covers both consensual and non-consensual acts. It may well be that the offences which are receiving such lengthy sentences are serious cases of non-consensual buggery rather than consensual homosexual sex.

The second exception is the sentence lengths passed on those convicted of indecency with children. Whereas the sentence lengths for the other listed sexual offences have increased, those for gross indecency with children have actually decreased steadily since 1980. One explanation could be that there may have been changes in the way the charge is used: it may be that those accused of the more serious cases of child abuse are now being charged with different offences such as unlawful sexual intercourse with a girl under 13 or buggery, which carry a possible maximum life sentence, rather than the two-year maximum carried by gross indecency (although the increase in sentence lengths for the former – from 31 to 38 months – is not great). It may also be the case that the increase in the proportion of offenders being imprisoned (up from 14 per cent in 1980 to 31 per cent in 1989) reflects a number of less serious cases receiving short custodial sentences, thus dragging down the average sentence length.

Nevertheless, the pattern remains: courts are increasing their use of custody in cases of sexual crime. It is true that this increase in the use and length of custodial sentences for sex offences could result from some change in the nature of the offences themselves, rather than from a deliberate hardening of attitudes on the part of sentencers. However, Lloyd and Walmsley's careful analysis of sentencing of rape between 1973 and 1985[14] shows that, in the case of rape at least, the harsher sentencing they found could not be explained in terms of an apparent increase in the occurrence of 'nasty' rapes which merited harsher penalties. There was a significant increase in the proportion of the rapes in which weapons and excessive violence were used, or in which victims were made to perform oral sex or submit to anal intercourse. More of the offences involved the victim being in the hands of the rapist for lengthy periods of time, and more of the offenders had previous convictions. However, Lloyd and Walmsley argue that: 'The increase in the level of sentencing . . . is evident whatever the nature of the offence.'

The increased use of custody appears to be a deliberate policy on the part of sentencers. However, the superficial impres- sion of judicial unanimity can be misleading. It is doubtful whether such a complex activity as sentencing, carried out by individuals so protective of their own independence as judges and magistrates, can be said to be driven by anything that can be described as policy. Given the relatively small number of sex offenders who come before the courts for sentence, few sentencers will pass sentence on more than one or two each year, and each sentence will be determined as much by the individual circumstances as by the sentencer's view of official policy.

There therefore remain inconsistencies in sentencing despite Lord Lane's sentencing guidelines. As Table 3.2 reveals, in 1980, before the Lane guidelines, only 12 out of the 337 rapists convicted by the courts (3.5 per cent) were known to have been given non-custodial sentences (ignoring the 'others', the majority of which may well represent offenders diverted at sentence to the mental health system). Despite the public perception, few rapists were escaping prison. In 1989, and despite Lord Lane's guidelines, 9 of the 476 rape offenders were still being given non-custodial penalties – a proportion of nearly 2 per cent. Either there are a surprising number of 'wholly exceptional' cases of rape, or some sentencers are still not heeding the sentencing guidelines.

Although the judges' sentencing practice may have changed to some degree, old attitudes die hard. Judicial thinking about sexual crime still clings hard to concepts which others have seriously ques- tioned, and these misconceptions still distort the sentences they pass. Thus, in July 1991, a rapist can be given a reduced sentence of three years because the woman he raped was, in the words of Mr Justice Alliott, 'a common prostitute and a whore'.[15] Similarly, in January 1992, a husband who raped his wife can be given only a suspended sentence by a judge who regarded the rape as 'a mis- placed attempt to get her to love you' and who argued that the 'psychological hurt' of being raped by an intimate was less than that which would result from being raped by a stranger.[16]

There is little to indicate that judges have come to appreciate the true nature of sexual crime and the damage that results from it. In 1982, Mr Justice Wild commented that:

Women who say no do not always mean no. It is not just a question of saying no, it is a question of how she says it, how she shows it and makes it clear. If she doesn't want it she only has to keep her legs shut and she would not get it without force and there will be marks of force being used.

These attitudes still exist. In December 1991, a judge sentenced two 16-year-old boys to supervision orders for their rape of a 15-year-old girl, arguing that they had regarded it as a 'prank'. Mr Justice Ognall added a stern warning:

If you are daft enough to muck about with young girls again there won't be a second chance.[17]

Efforts are now being made to counter such attitudes. In September 1992, and in a very unusual move, the Lord Chancellor's Department began showing groups of judges a video of a rape survivor (in this case, Jill Saward, victim of the 1986 Ealing vicarage rape) talking about her experience.

However, the attitudes are not limited to the lower echelons of the judicial community. In a case in 1990 where a 10-year-old girl was lured into a wood and buggered by a young man high on glue, the Court of Appeal voiced judicial doubts about whether sexual crime leaves survivors with any lasting effects:

It is of course impossible to say at this stage what, if any, psychological effect it will have upon her. One very much hopes none. That is something for the future which one can never know.[18]

They are also enshrined in official sentencing policy. In his guideline judgement on sentencing of incest offenders, Lord Lane listed among the factors to be used in mitigating sentence the girl's previous sexual experience and whether she had made deliberate attempts at seduction. Previous sexual experience has been held in statute to be not relevant in cases of rape; despite this, it is now a mitigating factor in cases of incest. The Lane guidelines also re-echo the old claims about men's need to relieve their sexual urges and their inability to resist sexual advances made by females. In Lord Lane's view, an 'ordinary' case of incest is one where the sexual relationship between husband and wife has broken down and the daughter becomes 'the object of the father's frustrated sexual inclinations'.[19]

Statements such as these indicate that although sentencing practice may now reflect more adequately the gravity of offences such as rape and child abuse, this change has come about more because of public pressure upon sentencers than because judges have come truly to understand the nature of the offences with which they are dealing. It is noticeable that despite their doubts about the seriousness of the impact upon the girl concerned in the last-mentioned case, the Appeal judges nevertheless acted to increase the offender's sentence from three years to seven.

CRIMINAL JUSTICE ACT: SPECIAL TREATMENT FOR SEX OFFENDERS

There is every reason to believe that the pattern of harsher sentencing of sex offenders looks set to continue. In part, this is a result of the continuing nature of the panic over sexual offending and the pressure exerted upon sentencers by politicians and the media. However, in part a further increase in sentence lengths is guaranteed by the strategy adopted by the Government to ensure the safe passage of the 1991 Criminal Justice Act.

The Criminal Justice Act was intended to introduce a consistency of approach to the sentencing process and to facilitate the diversion from custody of minor offenders. By creating an extended menu of possible sentences, including new sentences such as the combination order and the curfew order, Government hoped to persuade courts to rely less on the use of custody and more on community penalties. However, if only to sell such a policy to the public and, more important, to its own backbenchers, Ministers adopted a 'twin-track policy': while minor offenders were to be diverted from custody, those convicted of offences involving sex and/or violence were still to be imprisoned. Indeed, as the proposals passed from Green Paper to White Paper to Bill, and as Douglas Hurd was succeeded as Home Secretary by David Waddington and then by Kenneth Baker, the attitudes to offences of sex and violence became increasingly punitive. Ministers no longer simply argued that such offenders must be imprisoned; now they emphasized that they were to be imprisoned for even longer periods.

This process had two effects. First, it comprised a direct appeal to sentencers to increase sentence lengths. Second, Ministers allowed the introduction into the Bill of a method of empowering courts to sentence more harshly: the Government accepted amendments sponsored by Conservative backbenchers which provided courts with the powers to pass more lengthy sentences upon those convicted of offences involving sex or violence. Under Section 1 of the Act (which came into force in October 1992), backed up by Section 25, courts are permitted to sentence sex offenders to terms of imprisonment longer than would be justified by the seriousness of the offence if they consider it necessary in the interests of the protection of the public.

Sex offenders are singled out for particular measures elsewhere in the Act. An exemption is made to the rule that offenders can only be sentenced to a maximum of 60 days' attendance at a probation centre or activity centre to allow longer periods of attendance to be imposed on sex offenders. An exception is also made to the rules governing the operation of the new parole and after-care system: while the statutory period on licence after release will end at the three-quarters point of their sentence for most ordinary ex-prisoners, for sex offenders courts can ensure that the licence does not expire until the very end of the sentence period.

These proposals met with considerable opposition from homo-sexual campaigning groups when it was realized that the list of offences to which the measures were to apply included homo-sexual offences such as soliciting and indecency between men, while excluding, for example, offences related to prostitution. The subsequent campaign had limited success in persuading the Government to amend the legislation to remove offences relating to the crews of merchant ships, procuring, and living off the earnings of male prostitution from the list. However, in the debate on 20 February 1991, the then Home Office Minister John Patten refused to amend clause 25 of the Bill further to eliminate references to indecency and soliciting, and to prevent it being applied to individuals convicted of consensual sex with males aged over 16 but under 21. In this he was encouraged by a florid speech by Dame Elaine Kellett-Bowman, who argued:

> Sodomy is unhygienic, unhealthy, and still the major cause of the spread of AIDS. If some highly-paid actors form a group, flaunt their perversion, and wish to protect others from custodial sentences, that does not seem to me to be a good reason to soften clause 25, or any others, to satisfy their sensitivity for such persons.[20]

These changes are clearly important in singling out sexual offenders of all types for particularly punitive treatment by the criminal justice system. This may well communicate itself both to offenders and to the wider society. The legislative changes are an explicit recognition that sexual crime cannot be treated in the same way as most other crimes and demands particular adaption on the part of the criminal justice system. The changes also link sexual crime and violence in an unholy alliance, a linkage which many victims will regard as a true recognition of their experience but which many sexual criminals – particularly those convicted of fully consensual offences – will find offensive. Indeed, there is a danger that the changes will only deepen some offenders' sense of being victimized unjustly for what they regard as a natural and harmless tendency.

However, the changes will have more than just a symbolic effect. The sentencing changes will not in practice affect offenders who have committed serious sexual crimes; courts will probably continue to pass lengthy custodial sentences for those offences. The cases that will be crucially affected are those where offenders have repeatedly committed minor sexual crime – cases which in the past may have been treated relatively leniently. Courts will now be able to pass sentences which amount to preventative detention on such offenders.

What use the courts will make of this new power is a matter for speculation. However, if the power is used, the Government could be in conflict with the European Court of Human Rights. It is probable that Sections 1 and 25 of the Act are in breach of Article 5(4) of the European Convention. Although sentences of preventative detention are not illegal under European law, the case of *Van Droogenbroeck v Belgium* in 1982[21] established that recidivist offenders given such sentences are entitled to periodic reviews by a 'court' to determine whether they are still dangerous. No such mechanism is established under the Act, and other case law indicates that review by the Parole Board will not suffice.

The fact that a measure which probably breaches European law could be included in such a high-profile Act is evidence of the Government's eagerness to appear to be getting tough on sexual crime. Government must have been aware of the legal status of the measure when the Bill was going through Parliament. The case of *Thynne, Wilson and Gunnell v UK* in 1989[22] had been brought on similar grounds and had forced a change in the release procedure for discretionary (non-murder) lifers. Thynne, Wilson and Gunnell had all been convicted of sexual crime and were given life sentences. Despite repeated reviews by the Parole Board, their release had been blocked either by the Board itself or by the Home Secretary. The decisions were taken in private, and no reasons were given. Their victory at the European Court established the right of discretionary lifers to a more open and just system of determining release, with no right of veto by the Home Secretary. The safeguards enjoyed by sex offenders given life sentences are now much in excess of those enjoyed by life serving sentences for murder.

That a Conservative Government chose to include the measure in the Criminal Justice Act, though regrettable, is perhaps not surprising. The attitude of the Labour Opposition, however, is equally regrettable. Despite being advised by Liberty (NCCL) and the Prison Reform Trust of the questions over the legal status of the measure, the Labour Party decided that it could not be seen to be speaking up for the rights of sexual offenders.

PAROLE AND REAL SENTENCE LENGTH

The actual length of time a long-term prisoner serves in custody is only partly determined by the judge. A large proportion of it is determined by the operation of the parole and life sentence release procedures. Here, too, policy has become tougher for sex offenders.

Until the implementation of the 1991 Criminal Justice Act in October 1992, prisoners serving longer than twelve months were eligible for parole after one-third of the sentence, with automatic release usually coming at the two-thirds point. The decision about whether or not to release a prisoner on parole was taken by the Parole Board, who made an assessment of the potential risk the prisoner posed to the public. In the cases of more serious offenders, the Home Secretary exercised a right of veto.

Even before the Criminal Justice Act, it was clear that sex offenders were being denied parole far more frequently than other offenders. In 1989, 50 per cent of parole applications by sex offenders were successful. In the same year, 60 per cent of burglars, 70 per cent of thieves, and 74.5 per cent of fraudsters were granted parole. Even where offenders had been convicted of violence, sex offenders did comparatively badly: 61 per cent of those convicted of wounding, and 51 per cent of manslaughter cases were successful.[23] Only those convicted of robbery or of trafficking in drugs were denied parole more frequently. Moreover, those sex offenders who were granted parole were far less likely than other categories of offender to be successful at their first review. The effect of this policy was to ensure that sex offenders were either released without supervision or received only relatively short periods on parole.

It will come as little surprise that this restrictive policy towards the granting of parole for sex offenders is a relatively recent phenomenon. In many ways, it has mirrored the increasingly tough sentencing of those convicted of sexual crime. In 1981, not only were the average sentences being handed out to sex offenders shorter, but the approach to parole was more liberal. Sex offenders were granted parole in 53 per cent of cases; exactly the same proportion of applications by burglars were successful. As with sentencing, a similar pattern can be seen with other offences of violence: in the same year, 55 per cent of wounding and 56 of manslaughter cases were granted parole.

In certain respects, this pattern was part of a deliberate policy. In 1983, the then Home Secretary, Leon Brittan, announced in his speech to the Conservative Party Conference that he would not be granting parole 'save in exceptional circumstances' to those serving over five years for offences involving sex, violence or drugs. The impact upon the effective length of time served in custody by serious sex offenders was immediate. In 1982, the year before the new policy took effect, 28 per cent of parole applications made by those sentenced to above five years were successful. In 1984, that proportion had dropped to 16 per cent. Indeed, those figures hide the true extent of the change. The Home Secretary's policy did not rule out the granting of a short period of parole in some cases; in a later policy direction to the Parole Board, he explained that a period on parole of up to eight months was within his guidelines. The effect of the change was therefore to ensure that almost no first applications for parole were successful – in 1984, just one of the 75 first parole applications was granted – and to limit the availability of parole to a few months towards the end of an offender's sentence.

The Brittan parole restrictions were finally removed by Kenneth Clarke in July 1992 as one of his first acts as Home Secretary. No explanation was given for this move, which was simply made in the form of a Home Office press release. However, under the terms of the Criminal Justice Act, although the Home Secretary retains a formal right of veto over the release of all prisoners sentenced to four years or above, the Government had committed itself to a policy of not exercising that veto in cases where the sentence was shorter than seven years. The Brittan restrictions would have scarcely been compatible with such a policy.

Nevertheless, the Criminal Justice Act also empowers the Home Secretary to make binding policy directions on the Parole Board. There is therefore some likelihood of them being reimposed should the Home Secretary come under political pressure to do so. It was noticeable that within weeks of the removal of the restrictions on parole, one newspaper began a concerted campaign to tighten up on parole procedures. In a series of articles and features in late July 1992, *Today* highlighted cases of violent rape and sexual murder committed by offenders on bail, on home leave or on parole. Victims and their families were quoted as demanding further restrictions on bail and parole for sex offenders – calls that were backed up by the paper's own leader articles.[24] The campaign met with little apparent reaction from Government, but the effects of such media-led out-cries on individual parole and home leave decisions should not be underestimated.

The effect of the policy regarding sentencing and parole throughout the 1980s was unequivocal. Sex offenders were being sentenced to longer and longer of periods in custody. As Chapters 5 and 6 will show, that period in custody was likely to be spent in some of the worst conditions the British prison system had to offer, with little access to outside support and little oppor-tunity to address the reasons for their offending. Few sex offenders were being granted parole, and those who were tended to be those convicted of lesser offences. The more serious the offence, the less likely was parole, and the shorter would be the period of parole supervision.

The changes in the Criminal Justice Act have reversed that policy. All serious sex offenders will now spend considerable periods under supervision in the community. In addition, the prison-based sex offender treatment programme means that many of those offenders will have undertaken some sort of work to challenge their offending. The pressures are now on the pro-bation service to take responsibility for dealing with the per-petrators of sexual crime. But, as the next chapter will show, there are questions about whether they are ready to do so.

Chapter 4

Sex offenders and probation: a challenge ducked?

Despite all the panic about sexual crime, the sentencing statistics suggest that the probation service has scarcely increased its level of involvement with sex offenders. The increasingly tough approach of the courts towards the sentencing of sex offenders has meant that one-third of those convicted of sexual crime are now sent straight to custody. Of the others, around one-third are fined and a further fifth are either conditionally discharged or receive a suspended prison sentence. Less than 15 per cent receive a community sentence which involves supervision by a probation officer. The proportion of sex offenders placed on probation in 1989 remained at 12 per cent, exactly the same as it was in 1980. On those figures, it can scarcely be said that the probation service has responded significantly to the new challenge.

However, the figures vastly underplay the involvement of the probation service with sex offenders. Alone among the host of agencies involved in the criminal justice system, the probation service retains an over-arching responsibility for offenders from the start of the criminal justice process to the very end: from first court appearance to release from custody. Indeed, some argue that its responsibility begins earlier than that: probation officers are becoming increasingly involved in crime prevention schemes and in co-operation with other agencies such as social services and the NSPCC in joint child protection initiatives.

Even without these, probation service involvement with sex offenders is considerable. Probation officers work on panels making assessments about whether or not to prosecute or caution offenders. They run bail information schemes at Magistrates' Courts and bail hostels housing defendants awaiting trial. They staff the courts and provide magistrates and judges with pre-sentence reports containing assessments of offenders and recommendations as to sentence. They supervise a wide range of community penalties: probation orders (with or without conditions attached), community service orders, supervision orders, even money payment supervision orders for those who have been given financial penalties. They work with prisoners, either as prison probation officers or as outside throughcare officers, acting as a link with the world outside and helping offenders plan for their release. Finally, they supervise offenders who have been released from custody on parole or the automatic after-care licence introduced in the 1991 Criminal Justice Act.

The level of probation involvement with sex offenders is set to increase further as a result of the 1991 Criminal Justice Act. The Act places on the probation service an obligation to produce a pre-sentence report on all serious offenders (inevitably including almost all of those charged with sexual crime) convicted by the courts. It allows for the 60-day time limit for attendance at probation centres or the performance of 'required activities' to be exceeded in the case of sex offenders. It also requires that all those sentenced to over one year in prison will be on statutory probation licence after release, and in the case of sex offenders, allows for that licence to be extended up to the end of their sentence.

The effect of these changes will be to increase the number of sex offenders for whom the probation service has a statutory responsibility. This was confirmed in a speech to a tripartite seminar on 'The Effective Management of Sex Offenders' in late 1991 by John Halliday, Deputy Under-Secretary of State at the Home Office:

> The probation service's caseload of sex offenders will rise for two reasons. First, because of the expected increased use of non-custodial sentences for offenders at the lowest end of the scale, for whom public protection is not the paramount issue, and whose offending will be most appropriately dealt with through community-based programmes, rather than imprisonment, and – second – because of the substantially increased number of sex offenders on post-release licence. In 1990, 1190 persons convicted of sexual offences started probation orders and 150 community service orders, whilst at present about 400 sex offenders are on parole licence. Our projections of prison discharges are that 1700 offenders will be

released from custody annually of whom 700 will have been sentenced to four years or more and whose supervision period may extend over several years. Furthermore, we anticipate that to be successful, post-release supervision of sex offenders will normally be more intensive than for other kinds of offenders.[1]

The projections given by John Halliday represent a massive increase in the extent of the probation service's work with sex offenders. The Home Office has provided no specific estimates of the increase in the number of community orders on sex offenders which the probation service will have to supervise. However, the changes to the parole and after-care systems in the 1991 Criminal Justice Act will more than quadruple the number of sex offenders on licence. That represents a huge challenge to the probation service.

The changes in the Act and the range of tasks undertaken by the probation officers, in theory, render them key arbiters of policy towards sex offenders. They are able to influence decisions regarding prosecution and sentence, and to offer offenders access to treatment, either in the community or in institutions. So what has been the response of the probation service to the increasing level of concern about sexual crime, and the increasing number of sex offenders with whom it will have to deal?

STRUCTURE AND MANAGEMENT

Any attempt to evaluate the probation response is complicated by the fact that the probation service is a very devolved body. There are currently some fifty-five probation areas in England and Wales. Each is managed by a Chief Probation Officer accountable to a local Committee, an independent body largely made up of local magistrates and dignitaries. The policies and priorities of each probation area are decided by the Chief Probation Officer in consultation with the Committee. Although all the probation areas are ultimately accountable to the probation division in the Home Office, the Home Office merely lays down broad policy guidelines, rather than, for example, the detailed instructions issued by Prison Service Headquarters to prison governors. Each local probation area decides policy towards sex offenders according to its own needs and wishes; machinery to co-ordinate the approach of the probation service simply does not exist.

The problems engendered by such a structure are recognized in the Home Office, and the 1980s saw increasing attempts by Government to centralize policy-making in the probation service. In 1984 a Statement of National Objectives and Priorities (commonly referred to as SNOP) was published; it was the first Home Office attempt to set out in writing the priorities and policies it wanted from the service. In 1988, probation areas were required to produce 'Action Plans' for tackling offending by 17–20-year-olds. In 1989, the Audit Commission produced a report calling for the creation of a more tightly controlled service with clear objectives and a more consistent approach. The 1991 Government decision document *Organising Supervision and Punishment in the Community* confirmed this approach, seeking to create a probation service which operated within 'a centrally determined framework of objectives and accountability'. Finally, the implementation of the 1991 Criminal Justice Act in October 1992 was accompanied by the issuing of national standards for probation supervision. All these demonstrated the Home Office's anxiety to impose a centralized policy on the various probation areas. Despite this, local probation services still remain largely independent of central control.

It is worth mentioning that in this flurry of instructions from the Home Office, the proper probation response to sexual offenders was rarely if ever touched upon. There were attempts to standardize policy towards other specific groups, noticeably juveniles and young offenders, and, to a lesser extent, drug and alcohol abusers. However, sex offenders figured not at all. Indeed, some of the priorities set in SNOP and its successors militated against successful intervention with sex offenders. In particular, the down-grading of work with offenders in custody signalled in SNOP and the priority given to the supervision of statutory court orders at the expense of work with prisoners had a considerable impact upon probation officers' ability to intervene with the more serious sexual offenders.

However, probation policy is rarely in practice made by the management of the fifty-five different probation areas. Probation service culture is largely 'bottom-up', with individual probation officers or probation teams enjoying considerable autonomy of practice. The service has traditionally depended upon its ability to recruit highly motivated and educated staff, despite a relatively low level of pay. Probation officers have been encouraged to regard their role as a vocation or profession akin to medicine or law, whose practitioners brook little interference in their work. The legacy of the psychodynamic model of probation work, with its emphasis on the sanctity of the relationship between therapist and client, has also led to an unwillingness on the part of staff to allow management much scope for control of what they do. This tradition of autonomy on the part of the grass-roots staff has not been challenged by a management almost universally drawn from the ranks of former probation officers and educated in the same culture.

The absence of central control of policy is particularly crucial given the wide variation in the size and nature of the different probation areas. Policies adopted by a large, rural probation service may need to differ markedly from those adopted by a small, urban one. The pressures on probation officers in an area of great poverty or unemployment are very different from those in an area of greater affluence. Offending rates differ from probation area to probation area. The proportion of offenders with drug or alcohol problems, the number of burglaries or car thefts, and the sentencing practices of the local courts all differ and require a very different response from the probation service.

This problem is particularly acute in the case of sex offenders. Differences in the policies of different police forces and social services departments have produced wide variations in the number of offenders detected and prosecuted. These are magnified in turn by differences in the response of magistrates and the judiciary. The effect of these disparities is to ensure that the number of sex offenders dealt with by the probation service differs markedly from probation area to probation area. According to the Chief Probation Officer of Shropshire, in October 1991 there were 400 sex offenders being supervised by the Manchester probation service but only 25 scattered over the whole of Powys.[2] Mary Barker and Rod Morgan found an even wider range, between the 6–8 sex offenders on the probation caseload in the Channel Islands and the 518 in the West Midlands.[3]

AN EXPLOSION OF ACTIVITY

Given these pressures, the probation service's response to any issue is inevitably patchy and difficult to evaluate. Nevertheless, a clear pattern of probation response to the issue of sex offending can be discerned. In 1980, work with sex offenders was a very low priority for most probation services. In part, this was because of an inadequate appreciation of the seriousness of the problem. According to the Association of Chief Officers of Probation:

the received wisdom seemed to be that, with a few notable exceptions, sex offending was the product of impulsive 'lapses' resulting from abnormal circumstances (e.g. sickness of a wife) or of strange subcultural norms (incest in isolated rural communities). The effect on victims was hardly considered. The number of sex offenders supervised by the service was small and few of us had either the specialist training or experience to challenge the largely collusive supervisory relationships we maintained with perpetrators.[4]

Even among probation officers who recognized the need to tackle sex offenders' behaviour, there was a pessimism about how much could actually be achieved. During the late 1970s and early 1980s the probation service was undergoing a crisis of confidence about the effectiveness of its work. The probation service, along with the prison system, had invested heavily in the 1960s and 1970s in the rehabilitative ideal, the notion that it was possible to change individuals to ensure that they would not offend. By the late 1970s, disillusion was beginning to set in. The new pessimism was summed up in the 'nothing works' philosophy advanced by Robert Martinson in his short paper 'What works? Questions and answers about prison reform'.[5] Published in the USA in 1975, Martinson's conclusions were echoed in the UK in 1976 by the work of Brody[6] and the findings of the IMPACT study of Folkard et al.[7] The probation service was unable to demonstrate convincingly that its work really had a direct impact on reoffending rates.

By the late 1980s, some degree of confidence in the concept of rehabilitation was beginning to seep back into the probation service. The fierce rejection of the notion of rehabilitation had begun to wane: George Mair's careful examination of the debate shows the gathering weight of authority questioning – and rejecting – Martinson's arguments.[8] Further stimulus came from the high-profile attempts of workers such as Robert Ross[9] to document and sell effective treatment programmes from across the Atlantic. More particularly, the publicity accorded to the work of such figures as Ray Wyre, a former probation officer and now Director of the Gracewell Clinic, gave some confidence that effective work with sex offenders was possible.

By the late 1980s, the renewed confidence about the effectiveness of probation work, combined with a belated recognition of the need to respond to the challenge of sexual crime, was beginning to show results in the probation service. The explosion in activity in the field can be traced in a series of surveys of probation work with sex offenders. One survey was carried out by Carolyn Yates from Essex University in March 1989.[10] Between July and October 1990, HM Inspectorate of Probation implemented a thematic review, including a detailed examination of the work being performed with sex offenders in six probation areas.[11] Also in 1990, Leah Warwick surveyed work throughout the probation service.[12] Finally, Mary Barker and Rod Morgan carried out an evaluation of sex offender treatment for the Home Office in 1991.[13] The pattern of response revealed by these surveys is clear.

Superficially at least, there are signs of a tremendous growth in probation work with sex offenders. In March 1989, Yates found that twenty-one of the fifty-six probation areas then in existence (the City of London Probation Service has since been absorbed into Inner London) claimed to be running specialist programmes for sex offenders. By the time of Barker and Morgan's survey in 1991, that number had expanded to forty-one, with a further seven services planning to begin programmes in the near future. This trend has subsequently been borne out by a survey by the Prison Reform Trust of forty-seven probation areas which, in October 1992, found only one probation area claiming not to be running specialist programmes.[14]

However, the authors of these surveys expressed worries about how far this impressive level of activity will be maintained. Many of the schemes have become well-established models for the effective supervision of sex offenders in the community. The sex offender initiatives in Avon, Leicestershire, Nottingham, Oxford, and North East London have all established themselves as valuable and authoritative projects, trusted by sentencers and seemingly effective in reducing reoffending. However, these were not totally representative. The vast majority of the projects examined by the surveys were of comparatively recent origin: all but five of the fifty-three programmes identified by Barker and Morgan had been in existence for less than five years, and over a quarter had been in existence less than a year.

MANAGEMENT PROBLEMS

This explosion of activity is heartening testimony to the interest aroused in the probation service by the problem of sexual crime. However, there are major problems with which they will have to contend. First, as the surveys reveal, it was clear that the vast majority of the specialist provision of which management was boasting represented the fruit of grass-roots initiative unsupported by management. As the HM Inspectorate of Probation Report concluded:

> While some 'centres of excellence' have been created within the service, frequently inspired and led by middle managers or main grade staff particularly committed to such work, it is, nevertheless, the Inspectors' view that while some initial development may be grass roots led, the long term provision of such facilities and the support and supervision for staff is the responsibility of management and should be built into the official management systems of area and division. This was not always the case.[15]

Barker and Morgan echo this conclusion:

> All accounts of the development of sex offender treatment in probation suggest that the first initiatives are very much practice-led. In Avon, Hampshire and Nottingham, where programmes began in the form of groupwork over ten years ago, the initiators in each case seem to have been main grade officers who developed a particular interest in sex offenders. They ran the groups in their own time and only in the last few years have they begun to receive what could be called 'active' management support.[16]

The absence of effective managerial involvement and oversight was crucial to the operation of these initiatives. All the surveys found that the stimulus for the initiatives had come from the interest of the officers running them, and that the work had largely been undertaken in addition to those officers' normal duties. Relief from their normal duties or time off for training could only be achieved through the informal agreement of colleagues. This was a source of considerable strain. Management support was therefore essential in order to ensure the provision of adequate staffing and resources.

Unfortunately, those resources could not always be provided. The expansion in the number of sex offender programmes coincided with a crisis in probation resourcing. Funding for the probation services comes from two sources: the Home Office provides 80 per cent of the funding, with the remaining 20 per cent being made up by the local authorities in the area covered by the probation service concerned. Until the late 1980s, the financial control of probation area budgets had not been particularly stringent. However, the successive Criminal Justice Acts of the 1980s loaded an increasing amount of work onto the probation service. At the same time, the cuts in local authority budgets, and the governmental drives to increase efficiency and control public expenditure, placed an increasing responsibility on probation areas to demonstrate their cost-effectiveness. In particular, the introduction of cash limits for the probation service in the 1991 Criminal Justice Act, which took effect in April 1992, ensured direct Government control of the size of probation areas' budgets.

The relatively small number of sex offenders officially on probation caseloads meant that devoting resources to the provision of services for them was, for many probation areas, very difficult to justify. In 1989, only 1,081 (2.5 per cent) of the 42,000 offenders being supervised on probation by the probation service had been placed on probation for (indictable) sexual offences. The number of sex offenders on community service orders was even lower: 0.3 per cent. A further 0.6 per cent of probation orders had been given for indecent exposure. The coincidence of financial exigencies and other pressures on resources meant that few probation services were prepared to back their support for sex offender initiatives with money. So, Baker and Morgan discovered, only fifteen probation areas had been willing to recognize sex offender work as part of any officer's job description. Management's failure to provide resources to ensure time off in lieu had forced the closure of one programme which had been running continuously for fourteen years.[17]

The absence of effective managerial involvement with work with sex offenders had also made it difficult for staff to be properly selected and trained and for effectiveness of the initiatives to be assessed. If the culture of the probation service is resistant to management oversight and control, that is more powerful in the case of work with sex offenders. It has become axiomatic that sex offenders are 'different' from other offenders and that the work should only be undertaken by individuals who have extensive knowledge and training. The skills and knowledge acquired by probation staff in setting up and running sex offender initiatives has often far outstripped that of probation management. The ignorance of some senior probation staff about sex offending and sex offenders has served only to deepen their reluctance to supervise such work.

Some probation services, such as Manchester and Avon, which have a long history of work with sex offenders, had sufficient expertise among their staff to be able to provide training 'in-house'. Others, such as Nottingham, have even gone so far as to publish training packages for sale to other services.[18] Many other services have had to go outside the probation service to make use of Gracewell in Birmingham as a central training resource. The Gracewell Institute and the Gracewell Clinic were established in 1988 to provide a specialist residential treatment programme for sex offenders. Partly profit-making and partly charitable, Gracewell began offering both treatment for sex offenders and training and advice to other interested parties. Contact with the probation service has been particularly close, in part because of Ray Wyre's background as a former probation officer. According to Barker and Morgan, no fewer that twenty-eight of the forty-four services running programmes had sent staff on Gracewell training courses. Many others were making use of Gracewell literature in their work.[19]

The absence of formal management oversight has meant that little guidance has been provided about the theoretical base for the work. The Gracewell connection provided some degree of standardization in the treatment methods being used for those officers who have attended the training courses there. The training materials, such as the Nottingham pack, being increasingly made available are also being supplemented by the high-quality practice guidelines being produced by some probation schemes. Colin Hawkes of the North East London Sex Offender Project, for example, has formulated a set of standardized principles for the writing of pre-sentence reports on child sex abusers.[20] These attempts to exchange knowledge and foster good practice have been aided by the setting up in 1991 of the National Association for the Development of Work with Sex Offenders, a multi-disciplinary professional association intended to co-ordinate approaches across different agencies involved in work with sex offenders and to act as the focus for the development of good practice.

The lack of formal management involvement in the initiatives was most strikingly signalled by the finding of Leah Warwick's survey that only six probation areas had developed any policy statement about work with sex offenders. This apparent lack of management interest forced those running the programmes to rely upon their own resources and support systems. But, perhaps most important of all, the lack of formal management endorsement of the initiatives has exposed the tensions within the probation service about how far it should be engaging in work with sex offenders and what style of work that should be.

STAFF AMBIVALENCE

Despite the huge growth in the number of sex offender schemes run by the probation service, there is by no means unanimity within the service that this response is the correct one. A motion at the 1991 NAPO conference calling for the expansion of probation sex offender schemes and the diversion of minor sex offenders from custody was lost by 326 votes to 281. A motion expressing concern about the leniency of sentencing of offenders against women and children was passed with none against. In both debates, many probation officers expressed the view that sex offenders should receive custodial sentences. The same conference saw the passing of motions calling for the diversion from custody of offenders who are mentally ill and of abused women who kill their abuser. These motions hardly represent a ringing endorsement of probation intervention with sex offenders.

The attitudes displayed during these debates are clearly deep-rooted, and felt by many probation officers. However, they appear to strike a note of moral condemnation rarely otherwise expressed by probation officers about offenders. There are also problems with somewhat simplistic formulations of the feminist explanation of sexual crime which have been adopted at NAPO conferences. A motion passed overwhelmingly at the 1992 NAPO conference expressed the beliefs that 'men have full and total control of their sexual behaviour', that 'sexual offences are an abuse of power' and that 'all sexual offences are violent offences whether or not additional physical violence is experienced'. An attempt to extend this formulation to include an acknowledgement that women, too, may be the perpetrators of sexual abuse, or even that men can be victims of abuse, was also voted down by conference. The motion used a single appellation – 'sexual offences'

– to cover a huge range of different behaviours, from consensual homosexual offences or consensual sex between teenagers to rape and child sexual abuse. It also failed adequately to distinguish between offenders whose behaviour raises very legitimate worries about the protection of the public, and those whose offences raise far fewer concerns. Motions such as this underplay the complexity of the issue and can allow prejudice to flourish.

There is already evidence that some probation officers are failing to recognize or apply these distinctions. The Inspectors of Probation found that:

> Writers of [pre-sentence] reports did not always differentiate between the seriousness of offences, e.g. between one in which there was a clear victim and another involving consenting adults.

Such a refusal to address the question of the degree of risk posed by an individual sex offender is hardly conducive to the creation of a sensitive and rational sentencing process, and the condemnatory attitudes expressed by some probation officers, can only serve to feed the increasingly punitive attitude of the courts.

The culture of condemnation which exists among some probation officers, and which has been fostered by NAPO conference motions, carries with it grave dangers. It serves to undermine attempts by some probation staff to create specialist initiatives in an attempt to reduce the risk of sex offenders reoffending. The view expressed about prison staff by Monika Sabor, a senior probation officer working in HMP Usk, could equally well apply to some probation staff:

> There is still a view amongst some prison officers that sex offenders do not deserve to be helped.[21]

Nevertheless, these attitudes are representative of real tensions in the work of probation officers with sex offenders. The challenge posed by sexual offenders goes to the heart of the underlying – and in the minds of many probation workers, often unresolved – questions about the proper role of the probation officer. As Tony Morrison, chair of the National Association for the Development of Work with Sex Offenders, has argued:

> Within the probation service tensions can exist between the service's duties to its own clients, the offender, and its responsibilities to the victim.[22]

The traditional debate within the probation service about whether probation officers owe their primary responsibility to the offenders, to the courts, or to wider society is thrown into sharper focus when the offenders being supervised pose (or appear to pose) such a high degree of threat to society. The need to ensure the protection of society appears to require a more rigorous approach to probation supervision, an approach at odds with the culture of many probation workers. Such an approach has the strong encouragement of the Home Office. Home Office Probation Bulletin No. 14, for example, places probation officers under an obligation to disclose the nature of a child sex abuser's conviction to any potential employer, particularly where the employment will bring the offender into contact with children. This sort of instruction, while undoubtedly in the interests of the public, nevertheless creates tensions, as Tony Morrison has argued:

> There can also be tensions over the degree to which the service's response to sex offenders is felt to be at odds with its response to the rest of its clients by being tougher, more invasive and less concerned with the rights of the sex offender than his [sic] responsibilities.[23]

The current specialist initiatives appear to be split on the question of how far work with sex offenders is compatible with a more traditional, relaxed approach and how far it is necessary to be more rigorous in approach. Baker and Morgan report that many programmes are content to take offenders on a voluntary basis, where there is no court order to be enforced. Many schemes, however, adopt the 'tough' and 'invasive' style of probation supervision which Government is seeking to impose upon the probation service in the form of the new standards of supervision for all offenders. The introduction of these standards is currently being resisted by NAPO. Nevertheless, it is inevitable that the necessity of supervising a large number of serious and dangerous offenders on statutory after-care licence will force probation officers to consider more invasive and rigorous styles of working.

These tensions in probation culture and philosophy can leave probation staff who work with sex offenders alienated from their colleagues. On the one hand, they can be thought of as being on the side of the offender, as being almost 'quasi-perpetrators'. On the other, their rigorous, confrontational approach to sex offenders can be characterized as being unnecessarily punitive. This, allied to the lack of management support, can sometimes leave specialist probation staff demotivated and alienated.

FUTURE STRATEGIES: SPECIALISM v GENERALISM

The absence of close management oversight of work with sex offenders or of coherent statements of policy about how such work is to be carried out allows such attitudes and tensions to go unchallenged. HM Inspectorate of Probation was adamant about the need for change. In particular, they argued that there was a necessity for probation areas to identify a manager responsible for work with sex offenders and to develop a statement of purpose about such work. There was an important symbolic element in having such a statement, legitimizing and supporting the initiatives which had been established. A statement of policy was also necessary in order to provide consistent guidelines about the theoretical principles underlying practice, and to resolve difficult choices about priorities and responsibility. Finally, it was important to have such documents as an aid to co-ordinating a multi-agency approach, involving prison officials, social services, health authorities and those responsible for any local residential provision. For all these reasons, a written probation area policy should have been developed in every probation area by 1 October 1992, the date of the implementation of the Criminal Justice Act.

However, the response of probation areas to the Inspectorate's instruction to prepare a statement of purpose about its work with sex offenders was typical of the inconsistent approach of the probation service to central policy. The Prison Reform Trust's survey of forty-seven probation areas in October 1992 revealed that thirty-three (70 per cent) had produced or were producing statements of policy. However, fourteen (30 per cent) had no plans to produce any separate statement of policy towards sex offenders. Moreover, the quality of these statements of purpose was extremely varied. Many comprised simple two- or three-page descriptions of work already being undertaken. Some merely reiterated existing procedures to be carried out when probation staff were involved in child protection cases. Few provided the strategic and theoretical expositions of policy recommended by the Inspectorate Report.

Nevertheless, the probation area statements of purpose – together with other probation papers, such as the 1991 NAPO professional practice guidelines[24] and the Association of Chief Officers of Probation position paper[25] – do make plain that there are the beginnings of a coherent probation attempt to decide policy towards to the increasing number of sex offenders with whom it will be required to work.

However, as those strategy documents show, the probation service will have to face some hard decisions in formulating its policy. In particular, probation areas will have to decide whether or not the service they offer to sex offenders are best undertaken by specialist probation officers or by generic probation case-workers. At present, as surveys of the probation service have made clear, sex offenders are dealt with by a mixture of both specialists and generalists. Few probation areas have established specialist units which are sufficiently well resourced to be able to deal with all the sex offenders for whom the area has responsibility. Also, few of these units are able to provide the whole range of probation tasks: assessment and report-writing, probation supervision, and through and after-care. In practice, many of these tasks are performed by generic probation workers.

This issue divides the probation service. In theory, it follows from the belief that sex offenders present very different problems from those presented by other sorts of offenders; that they pose greater risks to the community; that their problems are more entrenched; and that work with them should only be undertaken by probation officers who have been specially trained. The dangers they pose require specialist assessment. The compulsive and entrenched nature of their behaviour requires an approach which differs from the usual attempts by probation officers to challenge offending. And the fact that so many sex offenders are skilled in denial and in minimizing their offences could trap unskilled and unwary probation staff into colluding with their distorted beliefs.

The development of specialist probation initiatives would have other advantages. Staff selection problems may be reduced: not all probation staff want to work with sex offenders; some probation staff will themselves have been abused in the past, and may therefore prefer to 'opt out' of working with sex offenders.[26] The cost implications of training would be much reduced. Specialist units would generate their own 'esprit de corps' and would therefore be easier to support and supervise. Groupwork, an essential part of attempts to break down offenders' patterns of denial, would be easier to arrange. Finally, monitoring and the production of research papers would be facilitated.

The advantages of a specialist response are undoubtedly compelling. HM Inspectorate of Probation concluded that while only 25 per cent of work with sex offenders being undertaken by the probation service was of poor quality, the work that was poor was overwhelmingly being performed by generic rather than specialist staff. However, it is noticeable that few of the probation area strategies have adopted a specialist approach. In many cases this is for simple, practical reasons. In some areas, the geographical size of the region and the relatively small number of offenders dealt with render any attempt to create a specialist unit impossible. There are simply too few offenders being supervised (or likely to be supervised) in many large, rural areas, and the distances such offenders would have to travel would be too great to allow for the creation of a specialist unit. In other cases, it would be a waste of scarce resources to try to create a sufficiently large specialist unit to be able to deal with all the sex offenders for which that area is responsible.

However, there are other, less immediate reasons why some probation services have resisted the temptation to specialize. Some services clearly fear the effect on staff morale of handing over the responsibility for sex offenders to specialist teams. The ACOP discussion paper talks of the dangers of the specialist approach breeding 'charges or attitudes of elitism'. It is also inevitable that some generic probation officers will have to take responsibility for working with sex offenders at some stage. Sex offenders may well spend a period residing in bail hostels or attending day centres. They may spend periods in prisons where it is difficult for specialist probation staff to maintain contact. It is important that generic staff retain some basic knowledge of sex offender work.

There is also an important symbolic message in the decision. Some probation staff are concerned lest the policy of placing sex offender work with specialists reinforces the popular prejudice against such offenders. Tony Morrison has argued against an approach which conceptualizes sex offending

> as being very different to other types of offending, thereby negating previous knowledge and experience in dealing with entrenched and anti-social behaviour. This leads to tensions

about how work with sex offenders fits with the rest of our practice . . . Perhaps, too, sex offenders are the one client group with whom it would be unacceptable for us to identify. In consequence we may need to keep sex offenders at a safe distance from us both at an individual and at an institutional level.[27]

A COMMUNITY RESPONSE

However, as well as deciding the shape of the service to be provided to sex offenders, probation areas are also beginning to address the need to develop relationships with other agencies working in the field. Probation's role in dealing with the perpetrators of child sexual abuse places a responsibility on probation officers to co-operate with a host of other statutory and voluntary agencies: the Crown Prosecution Service, social services, the NSPCC, police, prisons, and other agencies such as the National Children's Home and the Rayner Foundation. Thus, for example, probation officers are under an obligation to pass information about the release plans of a child sex abuser to the police and the local social services department. In some areas, these obligations are clearly set out. In others, they are not. Similarly, probation officers may be required to participate in case conferences in the aftermath of child abuse cases. The creation of the sex offender treatment programme in prisons will also require them to retain much more contact with offenders while in prison and to co-ordinate their release plans to take account of the treatment offenders have received while in custody.

Nor is this all. The incoherence of the probation response to many sexual offenders and the nature of the phenomenon itself have ensured that sex offender treatment is now the province of many of those outside the formal penal system. The days when sexual crime was deemed to be solely the province of the medical profession are long since gone. However, many doctors and forensic psychiatrists retain a deep interest in sexual crime. Some hospitals continue to offer in-patient and out-patient treatment to sex offenders. Many probation services make extensive use of specialist psychiatric input to inform their work with sex offenders: the North East London Sex Offenders project was begun as a collaboration between Colin Hawkes, a probation officer, and Eileen Vizard, a psychiatrist from the Maudsley Hospital in South London. Other, more questionable partnerships have been forced on a reluctant probation service: in

1986, Mark Witham, convicted of indecent assaults on young boys, was released from prison and despite the concerns of his probation officer sought drug treatment from a psychiatrist to curb his sex drive. This eventually went ahead when the objections of the Mental Health Act commissioners were overridden by the High Court.

It is not just medical agencies with whom the probation service increasingly has to liaise. Collaboration with the Gracewell Clinic has its problems, not least the cost involved: a week's residence for an offender costs in the region of £500. However, such collaboration perhaps foreshadows the sort of probation practice necessary if the strategy of the Government 'peppermint paper' *Partnership in Dealing with Offenders in the Community*[28] and the encouragement in the 1991 Criminal Justice Act for conditions of treatment to be attached to probation orders are to be realized.

The necessity of the probation service acting increasingly in concert with other agencies will pose immense strains on it. The probation service, like other criminal justice agencies, is not accustomed to partnership. In some cases, it appears that it wilfully seeks to avoid formal co-operation: money provided by three charities to Northumbria probation service to co-ordinate its services to sex offenders with those of other local agencies went instead to create a local probation specialist resource. The three charities had to repeat their donation in 1992 before an independent agency, the Derwent Institute, was founded to do the job. Nevertheless, the necessity of co-ordinating policies with outside agencies will prove a challenge to the probation service, just as the necessity of co-ordinating its own policies on sex offenders has done.

The probation service will also have to work much more closely with the prison system. The large numbers of sex offenders released from custody each year will impose great strains on the probation officers required to supervise them on licence. As Chapter 6 will indicate, the hope is that many of these offenders will have undergone a period of treatment while in custody. The effectiveness of that treatment may well depend upon the probation service's ability and willingness to liaise with the prison service. Liaison will also be particularly important in view of the indications that prison governors will be able to write conditions into the offender's after-care licence. Unfortunately, the Prison Reform Trust survey revealed that by October 1992, less than half of all probation areas had had any contact with the prison system over the issue.

The changes in the Criminal Justice Act will also impose a greater strain on probation services' access to residential accommodation. In the case of the most serious sex offenders being released from prison – many of whom will have been in prison for some time and will be required to spend many years on licence – there may well be a need to provide supervised accommodation in the community where their behaviour can be observed. Unfortunately, only three probation areas currently provide any specialist accommodation for sex offenders. In around a third of probation areas, sex offenders are disqualified from hostel accommodation: the after-care hostel in Middlesex, for example, is situated near a school and has a veto on sex offenders written into its planning permission. The Gracewell Clinic has had similar problems with its planning applications.

None of these problems is insuperable, but all impose considerable strains on a probation service which is ill-equipped to deal with them. Nevertheless, there are encouraging signs that, in some probation areas, the need to make provision for sex offenders has acted as a spur for the service to look towards a collaborative, planned approach to offenders. The seven probation areas in Wales have reacted to the economic impossibility of being able to provide an adequate service to sex offenders on an area by area basis. They have therefore formulated a joint response, including a specialist residential facility to serve the whole of Wales. That approach is providing the planned, co-operative style of probation practice which has always been missing from the service.

Chapter 5

A prison within a prison

The increase in the use of custody for sex offenders, together with the increase in the lengths of time they are spending in custody, has had a marked effect on the prison system. In 1981, there were just 1,110 convicted sex offenders in prison; by 1990, the number had risen to over 3,000. In 1981, sex offenders comprised 4 per cent of the sentenced prison population; by 1990, that proportion had gone up to 7 per cent.

With most offenders, an increase in numbers of that sort would not pose any significant difficulties to the prison system. However, sex offenders pose a very particular challenge to the prison system. The challenge is two-pronged: how best to protect offenders from attack, and how to employ the period in prison to reduce the possibility of reoffending. How the prison system has tackled these problems forms the subject of this chapter and the next.

A CULTURE OF ABUSE

It is commonplace for sex offenders to be on the receiving end of violence and abuse while in prison. That abuse takes many forms. For many prisoners and in many prisons, antipathy towards 'nonces' or 'beasts' is little more than an idea, one of those prison mores to which they automatically subscribe when they take on the role of 'prisoner'. Few prisoners do more than pay lip-service to the idea. However, some prisoners actively persecute those convicted of sexual crimes. Verbal abuse is ubiquitous, with threats and taunts forming the normal verbal backdrop for life as a sex offender in prison. Food is adulterated: mashed-up cockroaches are stirred into stew or potatoes. Tea is a favourite target: 'You can tell when they've pissed into it because it floats on top, oily-like.'[1] Prisoners also find more subtle ways to express their contempt. One sex offender reported to *The Independent* that he had been made to look 'ridiculous' by the haircut he had been given: 'They chopped part of it bald and left other parts of it long.'[2]

But it is violence and the threat of violence which sex offenders fear most. The number of assaults which are committed on sex offenders in prison is difficult to gauge. The Home Office does not record such statistics, and there is good reason to believe that many assaults would go unreported to staff or unrecorded by staff. However, sex offenders themselves are only too ready to give first-hand accounts of physical abuse. Attacks take place in the showers, in reception, in association, and vary in intensity from punches and kicks to stabbings or assaults with a favourite prison weapon: a PP9 battery wrapped in a sock. Sometimes sexual abuse is used as punishment: in 1992, Birmingham Crown Court was told of how a prisoner who had already tried to murder one sex offender then raped his cell-mate when he discovered that the latter had been convicted of rape.[3] In some cases, attacks are alleged to take place with the explicit or implicit assent of prison staff; sex offenders are pointed out and staff simply leave the prisoners to do what they wish.

Support for violence against sex offenders in prison has also come from outside the prison system. Writing in the *Sun*, the columnist Richard Littlejohn called for the withdrawal of protection from sex offenders in prison. 'Then', he wrote, 'they can get the kicking they so richly deserve.'[4]

This theme was taken up by Terry Dicks MP in a speech in the House of Commons in November 1990:

> It is strange that the most violent criminal in our midst – the child abuser or the sexual offender – gets 100 per cent protection when he goes to prison whereas another violent man, a robber, has to live in the prison community. Because other inmates might not like the sex offender or what he has done, we have to pull him to one side and protect him; but who protects the young kid whom he violated? Nobody. So why the hell should such a man be protected in prison?[5]

It is at times of riot or disorder when sex offenders are at the greatest risk of attack. The riot in April 1990 at Strangeways prison, Manchester, saw horrifying stories of abuse and torture of prisoners accused or convicted of sexual crimes. Many of the initial stories which appeared in the newspapers on 2 and 3 April, stories of hangings, castrations and as many as twenty deaths, fortunately proved to be exaggerations. However, evidence given at the trial of the Strangeways rioters in March 1992 confirmed that mock trials of sex offenders and savage beatings had taken place. Some prisoners had only escaped by feigning death. At least one sex offender had tried to commit suicide in his cell. And one man, Derek White, remanded to Strangeways and accused of eight offences of sexual assault on his step-children, had been so badly beaten that he died in Manchester General Hospital on 3 April.

Such attacks on sex offenders are not new. John MacVicar has written of similar attempts on the life of Ian Brady in the 1960s. Indeed, it is part of the established routine of prison riots: once you have secured control of the prison, the two immediate priorities are to raid the pharmacy for drugs and to beat up the nonces. However, the persecution of sex offenders is part of a wider pattern of prison traditions, and is a product of the basic culture of prisons themselves.

Prisons are very traditional places, and prison traditions are deep-seated and long-lasting. To a large degree, these are a product of the primarily working-class, male culture shared by prison officers and prisoners. They are also a response to the need of prisoners and staff to find a *modus vivendi* which allows both groups to survive the experience of spending long hours in a stressful, degrading environment. The differing characteristics of individual prisons – their age, physical layout, function, and so on – mean that the traditions and culture sometimes vary from prison to prison, and the older prisons, such as Dartmoor, Wandsworth, Brixton and Wormwood Scrubs, often exhibit wildly differing cultures built up over a period of many decades. But in all prisons there is a pecking-order among the prisoners: murderers and bank robbers are at the top, the run-of-the-mill offenders in the middle, and sex offenders are very much at the bottom.[6] The only variation between prisons is the extent to which the low status of sex offenders exposes them to violence.

The position of sex offenders at the bottom of the prison pecking-order is hardly surprising. To a large degree, it mirrors the attitude of society outside the prison walls. It is not unknown for sex offenders to be the object of attack in the community as well as in prison. Richard Blenkey, gaoled for life in October 1992 after the sexual murder of a young boy, had on two occasions been beaten up by the parents of boys he had abused.[7] In June 1992, a convicted sex offender and his family were driven from their Bristol council home by a fifty-strong gang of local residents armed with bricks and stakes, and crying 'get the pervert out'. One of them justified the action to the press:

> That evil pig should never have been allowed to move back into that house after he went to prison. We all knew he had been jailed for interfering with children. We hate his sort round here.[8]

It is also traditional in the penal system: in the eighteenth century, sex offenders were frequently stoned to death in the stocks. However, the antipathy towards sex offenders is particularly marked within prison. Prison culture is essentially a macho culture, a culture that places a high value on traditional male status and behaviour. In Trevor Hercules' revealing words:

> It was a man's world where only men lived, no women to make us soft and loving, no children to make us responsible and caring, just hard men, macho men, frustrated cocks who strutted around without hens.[9]

In this sort of atmosphere, attitudes towards sex are conservative. Any sign of sexual deviation from the norm is derided and seen as a sign of being less than male. Homosexuality is hated and feared. Prisoners and staff alike often refer to those identified as homosexuals as 'she' (this despite indications that a sizeable proportion of longer-term prisoners engage in some sort of homosexual activity while in prison[10]). Child abusers are also seen as non-male: Ken Smith records a prison officer in Wormwood Scrubs referring to two sex offenders as 'Henrietta' and 'Joan'.[11]

It is towards those who have been convicted of sexual offences against children that most hatred is directed. Child abusers are labelled 'nonces' and 'beasts' and have to endure the routine verbal and physical abuse meted out by prisoners and, sometimes, staff. Attitudes towards rapists are traditionally more ambivalent. Macho prison attitudes towards women share many of the myths which rapists employ, and claims that the victim consented carry more weight coming from rapists than from child abusers. Nevertheless, it is against the macho ethic to direct violence against a woman. Again, Trevor Hercules sums up the prevailing prison ethos:

We as men have a duty to look after and protect our women –
how can any people be proud if their women are abused?[12]

Rapists, too, are often the victims of violence: Frank Welton, a
London taxi driver accused of rape, was beaten in his cell within
a week of his initial reception into prison.[13]

However, the persecution of sex offenders is not only an
expression of moral disapproval of their crimes. The existence of
the prison pecking-order fulfils a deep emotional need. The hier-
archy among prisoners allows the vast majority of those in gaol to
feel that, however bad their circumstances, there are others who
are worse off. Sex offenders also provide a handy outlet for
feelings of anger and aggression for which there is no other
avenue of expression. Persecuting sex offenders allows otherwise
powerless people the illusion of power.

For the staff, too, the abuse of sex offenders has its advantages.
Many staff share the prisoners' view of sex offenders. One
attempt to recapture a wing during the Strangeways riot was
accompanied by the sound of prison officers beating their batons
on their riot shields shouting 'Beast! Beast!', a reference to the fact
that one prominent Strangeways rioter had a conviction for rape.
Staff also may allow the abuse of sex offenders for more practical
reasons. Some staff encourage the existence of the prison
pecking-order in the belief that it makes prisoners easier to control. The threat of abuse may allow them a useful source of power
over sex offenders who are trying to conceal their offences from
their fellows; unless they co-operate, prison staff will threaten to
disclose the nature of their conviction to other prisoners. While
prisoners are fighting among themselves, their aggression is also
being safely channelled away from the staff. For the staff, stig-
matization of sex offenders provides a useful safety-valve.

PROVIDING PROTECTION

The traditional response to the threat of abuse and violence has
been the use of Prison Rule 43. Rule 43 (or in the case of young
offenders, Rule 46) allows the governor to order the removal of a
prisoner from association. There is a general assumption that all
sex offenders automatically go on Rule 43: lawyers and police
officers advise sex offenders to ask about Rule 43 on reception,
and prison staff automatically assume that a sex offender will go

onto the Rule. The alternative – that sex offenders risk going on normal location to expose themselves to possible violence and abuse – is rarely considered.

The use of Rule 43 as the primary method of protecting sex offenders has meant that the increase in the sex offender population in prison has resulted in a similar rise in the number of prisoners on the Rule. In 1983, when there was a total of 1,415 sex offenders in prison, the number of prisoners on Rule 43 for their own protection stood at 632. By 1989, the figures were 3,005 and 2,438 respectively. Since then, the official statistics have shown a steady decline from that peak: by June 1991, the official Rule 43 population was only 1,789, a fall of over 25 per cent. By November 1992, the figure had declined to 1,539.

However, the impression of decline is misleading. Since the late 1980s, the Prison Service has begun to reclassify protected locations for prisoners needing long-term segregation as 'Vulnerable Prisoner Units' (VPUs). Prisoners in these units are no longer on Rule 43 and no longer appear in the official statistics. Thus, for example, G,H and K Wings in Wandsworth, which previously held some 280 Rule 43 prisoners, were reclassified as VPUs in 1992, thereby reducing the official figures by a quarter. By November 1992, there were 2,226 prisoners in VPUs, giving a total population on protected locations of 3,765.

By no means all of those prisoners were sex offenders. Those who have committed sexual crimes are not the only prisoners liable to violence and persecution by their fellows; informers, prisoners who owe money or drugs to other prisoners, former police officers, and those who are simply unable to function in the prison milieu also seek the protection of the Rule. These groups account for a significant proportion of the Rule 43 population. However, the Home Office's Adult Offender Psychology Unit have estimated that some 70 per cent of those on Rule 43 are sex offenders.[14]

Not all sex offenders automatically go onto the Rule. Offenders who have friends in prison, those who are physically large or have the ability to 'front it out', and those who are able successfully to conceal the nature of their offences from other prisoners may well be able to manage on normal location. However, a cursory reading of the statistics indicates that the majority of sex offenders do spend some period on protected location. Often that experience will be relatively brief: in May 1989, of the 2,274 prisoners on the Rule for their own protection, 491 had been there for less than one month, and only 372 for over a year. The majority of prisoners on the Rule had been there for a period between three and twelve months. That reflects the fact that Rule 43 is usually a temporary response to the prisoner's fears or threats made in a particular prison, most often the local prison where a sex offender is received on remand or immediately after sentence. It is in local prisons that the nature of the prisoner's offence is most likely to be known, either through local newspaper reports or through other prisoners appearing at the same court at the same time. Later in the sentence, prisoners can be transferred to where their offences are not known or to VPUs where they will no longer appear on the official Rule 43 statistics.

The rise in the Rule 43 population has had disastrous consequences for the prison system. In part, this has been the result of a confusion at the heart of the Rule. The wording of Rule 43 indicates that it is designed to deal with two very different situations. It reads:

1) Where it appears desirable, for the maintenance of good order or discipline or in his own interests, that a prisoner should not associate with other prisoners, whether generally or for particular purposes, the governor may arrange for the prisoner's removal from association accordingly.

2) A prisoner shall not be removed under this Rule for a period of more than 24 hours without the authority of a member of the board of visitors, or of the Secretary of State. An authority given under this paragraph shall be for a period not exceeding one month, but may be renewed from month to month.

3) The governor may arrange at his discretion for such a prisoner as aforesaid to resume association with other prisoners, or shall do so if in any case the medical officer so advises on medical grounds.

On the one hand, Rule 43 sanctions removal from association for the purpose of maintaining control over the prison, in the interests of 'good order and discipline'. On the other, the Rule allows governors to remove prisoners in their own interests. Within the prison system, these two distinct uses of the Rule have come to be known as Rule 43 Good Order and Discipline (GOAD) and Rule 43 Own Protection (OP). Nevertheless, their presence in a single Rule has caused these distinct functions to become confused.

The confusion between the use of Rule 43 as a security measure and its use to provide protection has led to the limited response of 'removal from association' – that is, removal from free and unsupervised contact with other prisoners – being reinterpreted to mean total segregation. Total segregation may be an appropriate response to the threat posed by a subversive prisoner to the safe running of the prison; it may well be necessary to prevent a prisoner who is trying to start a disturbance from contacting other prisoners. However, total segregation is not always necessary in order to guarantee the safety of a sex offender from attack. As Lord Justice Woolf argued in his 1991 report into the prison system:

> In the case of the vulnerable prisoner, on the other hand, it is accepted that any more separation than is necessary to protect the prisoner is undesirable. The object from the start should be to return the prisoner to association if this is possible.[15]

As a result, Woolf strongly recommended a rewriting of Rule 43 in order to distinguish between its two functions and to allow a more graduated response to the need to protect sex offenders from attack.[16]

This recommendation has not yet been followed. Instead, the Prison Service has continued with its traditional interpretation of the Rule as meaning total segregation. This interpretation inevitably requires prisons to run an entirely separate prison regime for prisoners on Rule 43. However, the general increase in the size of the prison population that has taken place since the late 1970s, together with the gradual reductions in prison officer working hours under the 1987 Fresh Start agreement, have severely restricted the prison system's ability to deliver satisfactory regimes for prisoners on normal location, let alone those on Rule 43. Moreover, the local prisons – in which the use of Rule 43 has been disproportionately high – are the very prisons that have been forced to absorb the majority of the prison overcrowding of the last ten or fifteen years. They are also the prisons in which the physical conditions are the poorest and in which the drain on prison officer time of providing prisoner escorts to and from court has been the greatest. These are the prisons that are least able to respond to the need to provide a decent quality of life for prisoners on Rule 43.

LIFE 'ON THE RULE'

The result of these pressures has been that the conditions and regimes for prisoners on Rule 43 have often been intolerably poor. Sir James Hennessey, then HM Chief Inspector of Prisons, undertook a thematic review of Rule 43 in 1984. He concluded:

Prisoners segregated under Rule 43 in local prisons tend to be held in the worst conditions and experience the worst regimes of all inmates, and for many the conditions are unacceptable.[17]

A prisoner quoted in *Social Work Today* described life on Rule 43 in one local prison:

There are about 220 inmates on the Rule. The unit isn't physically separate from the rest of the prison – just occupying part of a wing. Rule 43 prisoners have no access to the gym, have association on only one evening a week (and then only if they have work) and more limited access to education. There is only one workshop for 60 and just a few other jobs – so most convicted Rule 43 prisoners are 'banged up' 23 hours a day. It is this highly restricted regime which is the main problem rather than the expected abuse (or worse) although that does occur.[18]

Nor is this simply a problem confined to older, overcrowded prisons. A month after the opening of Belmarsh, the first purpose-built London prison in a century, one prison visitor revealed that two sex offenders had attempted suicide because of persecution and no Rule 43 prisoner had yet been able to receive education or visit the library.[19]

Even the Prison Service's own Working Party on the Management of Vulnerable Prisoners agreed that conditions for many Rule 43 prisoners were not acceptable. In their 1989 report, they concluded that:

The only real benefit which derives from being on the Rule is the physical protection from assault or intimidation which it provides for the prisoners concerned.[20]

The effect of such conditions on Rule 43 prisoners is clear. In 1988, Stephen Tumim found that one prisoner in Parkhurst, a top-security 'dispersal' prison, had been subjected to a regime of almost continual lock-up:

The inmate who had been in the unit for eight months said he was beginning to find difficulties in relating normally when he had visitors. Either he could not stop talking or he could not concentrate because he was distracted by the conversations all around him. His behaviour towards us, and the observations of the senior officer, tended to confirm this.[21]

The policy of locking groups of sex offenders up in squalid, punitive conditions for long periods of time seems almost perfectly designed to reinforce those aspects of their character and behaviour that will pose a risk to women and children after their release. The endless hours many of them will spend in their cells leaves them little to think about other than their offences and little to do other than masturbate to their fantasies. Moreover, the abuse to which they are subjected, and the conditions which they have to endure, feed into the feelings of victimization which so many of them express. For many of them, especially those who abuse children, their rejection from the world of the other prisoners mirrors their feelings of rejection from the world of adults outside prison. The effect is to reinforce their commitment to the societies in which they feel more comfortable: the world of other paedophiles and of children.

By forcing sex offenders to live together in a group, sharing a common culture of persecution and rejection, Rule 43 therefore inevitably fosters the development of rings of sexual abusers – rings which sometimes survive beyond the prison landings. Some sex offenders have reported that paedophile information is freely exchanged in prison, and that the court transcripts from sex abuse cases are circulated as pornography. Nor does the process have to be so overt. Just as important can be the mutual reinforcement of the sorts of myths about sexuality and offending that are so important to sexual abuse. In particular, the availability of pornography in prisons and the attitude of many male staff members can reinforce these beliefs.[22]

To a large degree, the squalid and restricted conditions in which Rule 43 prisoners are held are a simple product of the pressures upon the British prison system. The impact of over-crowding, poor management and under-resourcing has created a prison system which struggles to perform even the most basic functions; in 1991, it emerged in answer to a Parliamentary Question that Birmingham prison does not even possess a sufficient number of pairs of underpants to allow each prisoner a change of underwear every week.[23] It is hardly surprising that prisons that struggle to run one full and active regime are incapable of running two.

Nevertheless, there are other factors at play. First, the confusion between the protective function of Rule 43 and its quasi-disciplinary dimension has allowed some prisons to take a particularly punitive approach to Rule 43 prisoners. In some prisons, Rule 43 prisoners are held in the 'block', the part of the prison reserved for prisoners who have committed disciplinary offences. In Birmingham, for example, two researchers found Rule 43 prisoners being held in the block, three or sometimes six in cells that were designed to hold one or two.[24] Even in some of the most modern and well-equipped prisons, such attitudes persist. In Wolds Remand Prison, the privatized prison near Hull which opened in April 1992, Rule 43 prisoners were initially held in the block and experienced the same regime as prisoners undergoing punishment (they were subsequently rehoused in the prison hospital wing).

Second, many prison governors deliberately provide restricted regimes to prisoners on the Rule in order to encourage them to return to normal location. For governors trying to stretch resources and staff hours to the maximum, Rule 43 is an irritation. There is also a belief on the part of some prison staff that prisoners only opt for Rule 43 in order to get a better life than they would on normal location (a belief matched by a general misconception among prisoners on normal location that the nonces get better conditions than they do). If by providing only limited regimes they can persuade some prisoners to stay off the Rule, the drain on resources is reduced. If, as a result, they also need put less resources into regimes for the Rule 43 prisoners in the process, so much the better.

However, the poverty of life for Rule 43 prisoners is partly the result of the Prison Service's deliberate refusal to give priority to an improvement in conditions. The Government response to Sir James Hennessey's thematic review of Rule 43 was unequivocal: 'Improvements for Rule 43 prisoners should not take place at the expense of other prisoners in the same establishments.'[25] That statement echoes the reluctance on the part of many prison governors to devote resources to improving the lot of Rule 43 prisoners for fear of incurring the wrath of other prisoners and, to a lesser degree, staff. As HM Chief Inspector of Prisons found at Wandsworth:

> Senior staff all appeared very conscious of the need to improve opportunities for time out of cell for Rule 43 inmates but at a pace which would not provoke a reaction from the main prison.[26]

However, there is some official encouragement for improvements for Rule 43 prisoners. The Management of Vulnerable
Prisoners Working Party argued that improvements could be
achieved from within existing resources:

> The lack of provision may arise from a failure of management to
> recognize that the problem must be faced or from a lack of effort
> to arrange resources appropriately. We believe that, given the
> management will, some dedicated effort and a moderate stand-
> ard of imagination, much can be done to provide a decent stand-
> ard of life for Rule 43 (OP) prisoners even where accommodation
> is limited . . . Innovative approaches can ensure provision of
> positive regimes without necessarily using more resources.[27]

This argument has some force. Few governors have been sufficiently motivated to devote much attention to the problem of
Rule 43 and the need to improve the conditions for segregated
prisoners. Given the other demands on their attention – overcrowding, endemic industrial relations strife, and the constant
threat of escapes or riots – that is hardly surprising. The argument
that improvements in prison regimes can be achieved simply by
changing the way in which the system is run is an attractive one.
As Ian Dunbar has argued, much could be done to improve life in
prison by challenging the obsession of many prison staff with
security.[28] There are undoubtedly vast improvements that can be
made in the quality of prisoners' lives which do not require an
increase in resources, as the changes made in the light of the
Woolf Report indicate.[29]

However, the arguments advanced by the Working Party are
fuelled as much by a recognition that there will be no increases in
resources as by a genuine belief that all that is needed is imagination
and will. Indeed, they sound suspiciously like the thesis advanced
by the Prison Service during the introduction of the 'Fresh Start'
staffing arrangements, that the major obstacle to the creation of a
decent prison system was not overcrowding and under-resourcing,
but inefficiencies in prison management and staffing. Six years of
Fresh Start have done little to confirm that view.

A REDUCTIONIST AGENDA: NORMAL LOCATION OR VPU

Rather than attempting to improve conditions for prisoners on Rule
43 at local prisons, the Prison Service has concentrated its efforts on

reducing the numbers of prisoners at locals seeking the protection of the Rule. That has been done by two means: by attempting to restrict prisoners' access to Rule 43, thereby forcing them onto normal location, and by the development of a system of VPUs. These were the strategies articulated in the Management of Vulnerable Prisoners Working Party, and were later amplified by means of a Circular Instruction to governors in 1990 (itself amended the following year in the light of the Woolf recommendations).

In the Circular Instruction (26/90), governors were encouraged to make greater use of their power to refuse Rule 43 to a prisoner who requested it. Any prisoner whose fears were likely to prove groundless or who could possibly manage on normal location was to be refused segregation. In practice, governors had been reluctant to refuse protection. In part, this was out of habit, and because it would cause less trouble in the short term. However, many governors also expressed fears that should a prisoner who had been refused Rule 43 be subsequently attacked, they would be held legally liable. Indeed, one such case, *Porterfield v Home Office*, was brought in March 1988 by a prisoner who had been attacked; although the case was eventually lost, the principle of governors' liability for decisions relating to Rule 43 was established. Much of the Circular Instruction was therefore devoted to instructing governors on how to avoid the legal consequences of refusing protection.

The encouragement given to governors to refuse Rule 43 may well stimulate the development of schemes to facilitate the return to normal location of prisoners who had previously been on the Rule. Prisons have for many years operated informal schemes that allow vulnerable prisoners the chance of life on normal location, usually by transfer to a prison or a wing where they and their offences are not known. However, the Prison Service psychologist David Thornton has described one formal arrangement between prisons in the South West in the early 1980s, where sex offenders were routinely transferred between prisons and where they were coached in the lies they should tell when they were questioned about the nature of their offence.[30] In some cases, prisoners were even given new prison records and numbers.

Unsurprisingly, the policy of encouraging sex offenders to conceal the true nature of their offences has come in for considerable criticism. Many critics have argued that giving official sanction to lie about offences will only reinforce sex offenders' tendency towards denial. The Woolf Report concluded:

We agree with the Prison Reform Trust that to encourage prisoners, in effect, to lie about their offences in order to survive on normal location, is no solution to this problem. We recognise the reasons for this advice being given. These prisoners can benefit if the nature of their offence is not known. However, we consider it wrong for a service, whose purpose is to assist the prisoner to lead a law-abiding life in custody and after release, to encourage prisoners to conceal the true nature of their offences. It should be possible for the Prison Service to deal with this problem in a more satisfactory manner.[31]

Formal schemes of the sort operated in the South West appear now to have been discontinued. Nevertheless, the encouragement given to governors in CI 26/90 to refuse Rule 43 will inevitably force sex offenders to conceal their offences from their fellow prisoners.

The second arm of the Prison Service policy, the development of the VPU system, took place largely on an ad hoc basis in the late 1980s. Self-contained wings or units were identified as suitable for prisoners on Rule 43 and converted for use as VPUs (although this did not always involve any extra resources). VPUs are usually run almost as prisons within a prison. Prisoners in VPUs often have their own workshops and education classes, and they exercise and associate separately from prisoners on other wings. The regimes in VPUs usually mirror those offered to prisoners in the rest of the prison. However, where VPUs are sited in local prisons, the stability of the population in the VPU and the belief on the part of staff that VPU prisoners pose fewer threats to security than their peers, often enable a more relaxed and liberal regime to be run in the VPU than in the rest of the prison. Where this happens – as it did in Bristol until the 1990 riot and currently in Wandsworth – it can often be a source of resentment for other prisoners.

As in the case of many specialized prison facilities, no formal statement of purpose exists for VPUs; however, according to the Working Party, they are intended for:

a relatively small number of medium- and long-sentence prisoners – mainly sex offenders and child abusers – who will fail all attempts to survive on normal location and who will need to remain in a protected environment until their discharge, while having the benefit of the facilities available to other medium- and long-term prisoners.[32]

By the early 1990s, the development of VPUs had outstripped this limited definition of purpose. VPUs became the accepted method of providing protection for sex offenders, and by the end of 1992 there were VPUs at eighteen different prisons. Former Rule 43 units, such as that at Wandsworth, were renamed VPUs. New prisons, such as Littlehey, Full Sutton and Whitemoor, were used to house prisoners who had been on the Rule. Long-planned changes of use, such as Albany's change of status from dispersal to training prison in 1992, were seized upon as opportunities for expanding the number of VPU places. Even the riots of 1990 – riots which affected twenty-seven prisons – were used to convert two Young Offenders' Institutions, Whatton in Nottingham and Usk in South Wales, into VPUs, taking prisoners mainly from prisons damaged in the riots.

This sudden expansion distorted the regional distribution of VPUs around England and Wales. The siting of VPUs had been linked to the regional system of prison management. England and Wales was divided into four geographical regions, each of which had at least one VPU: Stafford in the North, Gartree in the Midlands, Bristol and Dartmoor in the South West, and Albany and Rochester in the South East. In addition, there were three national VPUs: at Maidstone, Channings Wood and Wakefield. However, the disappearance of the old regional structure in the management reorganization of 1990 meant the end to a planned VPU distribution. The expansion of the system therefore took place in a piecemeal manner.

The development of the VPU system did not always benefit the prisoners. Little thought was given to the need of the offenders to be near their family bases, a principle repeatedly stressed in the Woolf Report. The expansion of the VPU at Albany on the Isle of Wight was particularly unpopular with prisoners, many of whose families had to make the difficult journey from London. The siting of a VPU at Dartmoor was equally unpopular. As the next chapter will show, this is a problem that is likely to worsen with the advent of the new sex offender treatment initiative.

Moreover, many VPUs suffered from the same scarcity of resources as Rule 43 units. When Sir James Hennessey's successor as Chief Inspector of Prisons, Judge Stephen Tumim, visited Stafford, a Category C training prison, he found that in the VPU:

The majority of inmates had no work, inadequate education provision and more often than not, no association . . . It was noticeable that the Unit, being in a sub-basement, was short of natural light and inmates were unable to go outside the wing apart from going to visits or to undertake PE. If inmates are to remain in this accommodation, the worst in the whole prison, then they should be given opportunity for more activities off the wing, e.g. attending classes in the education block, or attending services and sessions in the Chapel.[33]

TACKLING PREJUDICE

The Prison Service strategy, combining attempts to keep as many sex offenders as possible on normal location with the provision of long-term protection for the rest, has been much criticized. In particular, the Prison Reform Trust has argued the Prison Service strategy failed to address directly the real problem: the prison pecking-order. The reliance on total segregation, the Trust argued,

> in many ways institutionalises and even perpetuates the persecu-
> tion of sex offenders. It provides prisoners with a legitimised
> target for their frustrations and anger. As the Chief Inspector of
> Prisons has said, the existence of Rule 43 is proof that 'the Prison
> Service accepts this prejudice against the weak and inadequate'.[34]

This argument was echoed in evidence submitted to the Woolf Inquiry by the National Association of Probation Officers and the Parliamentary All-Party Penal Affairs Group, among others.

As these critics argued, the targeting of sex offenders for abuse is not inevitable. While not unique to the British prison system – persecution of sex offenders is a feature of prisons in Canada and the USA – the need for total segregation is almost unknown in European jurisdictions outside the UK.[35] Nor is segregation always necessary even in British prisons. Some British prisons have had considerable success in integrating sex offenders into their populations without violence and persecution, and also without lies and cover stories. Prisons like Grendon and Wakefield have a long history of tolerance of sex offenders, and newer prisons such as Littlehey and Leyhill had followed in their wake. It is these initiatives which should form the model for Prison Service policy.

This policy also has the support of the Woolf Report. Woolf's new formulation of Rule 43 would allow the sort of graduated response to the threat of persecution that would permit a gradual integration of sex offenders. At Littlehey, sex offenders had been housed in a separate wing, but had been gradually mixed with other prisoners in workshops and education classes – that is, in structured environments where close supervision was possible. It had then been possible to move some sex offenders into normal wings.[36] It is noticeable that even bastions of tradition such as Wandsworth are now considering a similar approach.[37]

However, as Woolf recognized, the process of integration would not be easy. It would be naive to assume that the doors of G, H and K wings at Wandsworth could be thrown open overnight without tragic consequences. Integration would require caution and commitment. Staff would need to be vigilant for any signs of abuse. Governors would have to be willing to react to persecution by disciplining the perpetrator, rather than – as so often – by moving the victim. Prisoners' attitudes would need to be challenged, but with tact and sensitivity: at Littlehey, the publicity given to the success of the integration scheme produced a backlash among many of the non-sex offender population, who found themselves having to justify their tolerance to their peers and explain to worried families what they were doing in a 'sex offenders' prison'. At one point, the Governor found it necessary to write an open letter to *The Times* explaining that not all prisoners at Littlehey were sex offenders.[38]

Moreover, the process of integration would depend upon the more general process of reform proposed in the Woolf Report. Fairer and more just treatment of prisoners would lower the level of anger and frustration for which persecution of sex offenders is such a tempting outlet. Similarly, purposeful and active regimes would be an outlet for energy and liberal regimes would give potential persecutors something to lose by their misbehaviour. The smaller prison units or wings proposed by Woolf – no unit should be larger than seventy prisoners – would enable closer supervision and the range of specialized regimes these units could offer would enable more flexibility in placement of prisoners.

Given these reforms, integration of sex offenders is possible. Not only would this ensure that sex offenders in prison would be adequately protected and able to lead a relatively normal prison life, but it would also tackle that other consequence of the segregation of sex offenders – holding offenders in conditions which increase, rather than reduce, the likelihood that they will commit further offences. It is the Prison Service's efforts to tackle the likelihood of sex abusers reoffending to which we turn next.

Chapter 6

Treatment in prison: order out of chaos

If the need to protect sex offenders from attack has long been recognized by the Prison Service, the need to address the reasons for their offending has only recently been acknowledged. The response of the Prison Service to the growing number of sex offenders in prison was initially focused principally on their need for protection. The report of the Management of Vulnerable Prisoners Working Party considered only the future of Rule 43. Neither it nor any other Prison Service document prior to the Strangeways riot mentioned issues relating to treatment.

POLICY PRE-STRANGEWAYS

This failure to address the core problem of sex offending was in part a result of the structural problems underlying the British prison system. The increase in the prison population during the 1970s and 1980s, the crumbling buildings and degrading physical conditions, the grumbling industrial relations unrest and the series of riots and disturbances all made it almost impossible to effect the sort of strategic planning necessary to implement a coherent response to sex offending. A prison system which, in many cases, was even failing in its basic duty to produce prisoners in court in time for their trials hardly had time to worry about such complex and difficult issues as sex offending.

But the failure of the Prison Service in the 1980s to devise a co-ordinated policy to provide treatment for imprisoned sex offenders also emerged from deeper causes. Throughout the history of the British penal system, there has been a fundamental debate about the purpose of imprisonment. Successive genera- tions of prison administrators have argued as to whether their role is to seek the rehabilitation of offenders, deterrence through punishment or mere containment. Prison policy has oscillated between these ideals, with idealistic attempts at rehabilitation repeatedly failing to live up to the claims of their proponents, leaving the field open for the proponents of punishment or containment. The mid-nineteenth century attempts at rehabilitation through the penitentiary and silent systems gave way to the explicitly punitive system endured by Wilde. The borstal system, established in the early years of the twentieth century, was the embodiment of the reforming ideals of Alexander Patterson; these in turn were replaced by the ideal of the 'short sharp shock' in the early 1980s. Punishment succeeded reform; reform succeeded punishment.

Throughout the late 1970s and the whole of the 1980s, the prison system was sharing in the general disillusion with the rehabilitative ideal. The dominance of rehabilitation as the central purpose of the penal system in the 1960s – a period which saw not just the rapid growth of the probation service but also the establishment of Grendon prison on a therapeutic community model – had shown little in the way of positive results. There was little sign that the prison system's new approach to dealing with offenders was showing any reduction in the recidivism rates. Prisons were being rocked by a series of riots, most notably the Hull riot of 1976. The 'nothing works' philosophy had had its effect on the prison system as well as on the probation service. By 1979, the May Committee of Inquiry into the prison system was reporting a complete loss of confidence in the possibility of imprisonment achieving the reform of the offender. Instead, May proposed that the aim of the prison system should merely be to provide 'positive custody' rather than to attempt to reform.[1] In the ideological climate of the 1980s, the prison system was not fertile ground for the proponents of sex offender treatment.

In a system which provided no official encouragement for attempts at rehabilitation and which was failing even to deliver the basic care for prisoners, the wonder is that any attempts at sex offender treatment were possible. Nevertheless, despite all the problems, some initiatives survived, and even flourished, during the 1980s. In June 1990, the then Deputy Director of the Prison Service, Brian Emes, was able to report to the Woolf Inquiry that sex offenders were being offered treatment in some 63 of the 125 prisons in England and Wales.[2]

However, Brian Emes's claim should be treated with some caution. The basis of the Prison Service's figures has not been disclosed: only one year earlier, the Home Office's response to a Parliamentary Question had strongly indicated that, in fact, the Prison Service had no idea which prisons were actually offering treatment. It appears that Mr Emes was basing his claim on a short Prison Service questionnaire and the results of research carried out by a former probation officer, Malcolm Cowburn, for his MPhil thesis – research which has never been published in full.[3] The precise nature of the work being undertaken at these prisons is unclear: the figures could well include counselling being offered on an occasional basis by individual prison staff alongside established and structured initiatives such as Grendon prison and Wormwood Scrubs Hospital Annexe.

These initiatives exhibited very similar features to those undertaken in the probation service. Like probation initiatives, the quality and longevity of the treatment programmes were very variable. As the Home Secretary admitted in a speech to the Prison Governors' Conference in November 1990:

> Up to now the provision [for the treatment of sex offenders] has been unco-ordinated, dependent upon individual initiatives, and inconsistent in approach – and it has not been properly evaluated.

In part, the unco-ordinated approach to sex offender treatment was the result of the structure of Prison Service management. Responsibility for sex offenders did not rest with any specific part of the Prison Service. One 1988 memorandum concerning sex offender treatment had to be circulated to thirteen different sections within the Home Office.[4] However, the absence of any attempt to co-ordinate sex offender treatment by the Prison Service meant that treatment initiatives were undertaken in a piecemeal manner. Initiatives would spring up largely because of the interest of a particular individual, and would rarely outlast that individual's departure. The programme in the late 1980s in Maidstone's Thanet wing collapsed immediately after the departure of the probation officer who founded it; no other staff had the motivation or time to take it over and, in any event, no one else in the prison knew exactly what she had been doing. The treatment model used would vary widely, dependent merely on the theoretical perspective (if any) of the individual concerned. Almost no training was available, and individuals were left to search for training materials from whatever source they could find. Few of the initiatives were ever subject to monitoring, and the results were seldom published or evaluated.[5]

Moreover, because the initiatives functioned largely outside official policy, they were at the mercy of changes imposed by an unsympathetic management. Grendon prison, opened in 1962 and run since that time on therapeutic community lines, began to specialize from a very early date in dealing with prisoners who had been convicted of crimes involving sex or violence. Despite the respect and admiration it has gained outside the Home Office,[6] Grendon has always been unpopular within the prison system. As a result, the Grendon regime has consistently been threatened by changes in staffing and population imposed by Prison Service management. The decision in 1987 to impose a VPU on Grendon was contrary both to the wishes of the staff and the ethos of the prison: Rule 43 had never been allowed in Grendon. Managers at Grendon have constantly been under pressure to sacrifice the therapeutic groupwork fundamental to the Grendon style so as to improve the output of Grendon's industrial workshops and to enable the staffing ratios to be cut.

If, in Grendon's case, none of these threats has had a significant long-term effect on the prison's regime, the same cannot be said of the other major pioneer of sex offender treatment in the prison system. Established in 1972, Wormwood Scrubs' Hospital Annexe was, with Grendon, for many years the last outpost of the rehabilitative ideal in the prison system. Whereas Grendon catered for a mix of sex offenders and violent or psychiatrically disturbed prisoners, the Annexe concentrated on those it regarded as addicts: prisoners addicted to alcohol, drugs, gambling or abusive sex. However, the introduction of the Fresh Start staffing arrangements in 1987, with the consequent cut in prison officer hours, severely undermined the regime. In early 1989, a large number of prisoners were transferred into the Annexe who, according to the probation staff working there, were entirely unsuitable for it. In the chaotic months that followed, the Annexe's founder, Dr Maurice White, resigned and the senior probation officer, John Hedge, withdrew his staff. Although the treatment groups later resumed, they were significantly fewer in number and prisoners began to spend much longer in their cells.[7]

The absence of any coherent attempts at sex offender treatment in British prisons was in stark contrast to jurisdictions abroad. During the 1980s, treatment initiatives for sex offenders were introduced in Canada, New Zealand and a number of states in the USA. The existing initiatives in the Netherlands and in Scandinavia were also expanded. In these jurisdictions, in contrast to Britain, work undertaken was co-ordinated and vigorously evaluated, with the results being published.

PRESSURE FOR REFORM

By the end of the 1980s, the Government was coming under pressure to develop a policy on sex offender treatment. The general reversion towards the concept of rehabilitation which had been affecting the probation service had begun to have a similar impact on the prison system. At the same time, the evidence of the extent of sexual crime began to increase. High-profile campaigns in favour of sex offender treatment were mounted by pressure groups such as the Prison Reform Trust and the Suzy Lamplugh Trust, the latter all the more powerful because its moving spirit was Diana Lamplugh, whose daughter Suzy had disappeared, presumed murdered by a sex killer. Other interest groups, such as the Gracewell Institute, began to make much of their alleged success in preventing recidivism. These campaigns inevitably attracted support from other liberal pressure groups. However, they also offered the seductive prospect of a solution to the problem of sexual crime and allowed Government and penal reformers alike to show that they were taking seriously the need to protect women and children from abuse.

Once again, the Strangeways riot of April 1990 and the Woolf Inquiry which followed it was crucial in focusing Home Office attention on the need to reassess its approach to the treatment of sex offenders. The necessity of reconsidering the use of Rule 43 concentrated attention on the consequences of the Home Office's failure to make specialist provision for tackling offending behaviour. Evidence presented to the Woolf Inquiry emphasized that the policy of, in effect, creating sex offender ghettos without providing treatment only served to increase the danger of sex offenders reoffending after their release. As the Prison Reform Trust argued:

Even if one does not believe that offenders' behaviour can be changed for the better by their prison experience, one must accept that it can be changed for the worse. There is an obvious danger in simply locking up large numbers of sex offenders in a single unit – the danger of the development of an atmosphere where sex offenders reinforce each other's aberrant beliefs and learn from each other's sexual repertoires. Specialist provision may help to counter this tendency and challenge those beliefs.[8]

These arguments were echoed in the Woolf Report itself:

We also propose that more attention should be given to treatment. Many of those who gave evidence, including the Prison Reform Trust and the National Association of Probation Officers, stressed the unsatisfactory situation which results from our current approach to sex offenders. All too often they are left with no other company than that of another sex offender.

We recognize that when Rule 43 prisoners are subject to assaults or worse, this makes them feel, with justification, that they are the victims. It focuses their attention on their own condition and away from what they have done to *their* victims. This situation cannot be allowed to continue. Those offenders need to be assisted to avoid offending again. They must be required to confront their criminal conduct.[9]

Even before the publication of the Woolf Report in February 1991, this pressure had begun to have effect. The Prison Service management reorganization had at last located responsibility for the treatment of sex offenders in a single department – the Department of Inmate Programmes, headed by the former Deputy Director General, Brian Emes. He, together with the head of DIP2 section, Eddie Guy, organized a conference of prison staff working with sex offenders. This was held at the Prison Service College between 30 January and 1 February 1991. The proceedings of this conference were published by the Prison Service in July 1991 as *Treatment Programmes for Sex Offenders in Custody: A Strategy* and formed the basis of the treatment initiative announced on 7 June 1991 in a speech to the Suzy Lamplugh Trust by Kenneth Baker, then Home Secretary.

HOME OFFICE TREATMENT STRATEGY

The Home Secretary proposed a new initiative for the treatment of imprisoned sex offenders. All sex offenders sentenced to four years or above were to be assessed immediately after sentence in order to determine which of them were most in need of treatment. This assessment was to be carried out at one of six prisons in England and Wales: this list originally comprised Albany, Dartmoor, Full Sutton, Maidstone, Wakefield and Wandsworth. Young offenders would go to Aylesbury for assessment and women to New Hall or Styal. The assessment process would take account of offenders' previous history and current offences, their social and sexual functioning, and their willingness to participate in the programme. This would involve the use of penile plethysmographs, instruments employed as a means of identifying offenders' patterns of sexual arousal.

Once offenders had been assessed and had consented to parti-cipate in the programme, they would be assigned to one of two types of treatment: the core or the extended programme. Core programmes would be run either at the assessment prison or at any of another fourteen institutions. The list given in the July 1991 Strategy Document includes in addition to the assessment prisons: Littlehey, Channings Wood, Featherstone, Risley, Usk, Wayland, Whatton, Grendon, Wormwood Scrubs, Swinfen Hall and Feltham. Those prisoners assessed as requiring the extended programme would be treated at one of the original assessment prisons. In addition (although this was nowhere mentioned in the Strategy Document), some prisoners assessed as requiring treat-ment would not be assigned to the programme in order to pro-vide a control group against which the success of the initiative could later be measured.

The precise content of the core and extended programmes was to be drawn up by working parties of prison staff. The core programme was to concentrate on sex offenders' attitudes. According to the Strategy Document, it aimed to

> tackle offenders' distorted beliefs about relationships, enhance their awareness about sexual offences on the victim, and seek to get inmates to take responsibility for and face up to the consequences of their own offending behaviour. The pro-gramme will also get inmates to develop relapse prevention strategies, identifying the nature of their offence cycles and how high-risk situations can be avoided.[10]

This programme would be run primarily by non-specialist prison staff, often uniformed prison officers or probation officers, with support from prison psychologists. Offenders would usually attend two groups a week over a period of fifteen to twenty weeks.

The core programme itself was developed by a working party of prison staff over the last few months of 1991. It is explicitly based in the cognitive behavioural tradition and draws mainly on the work of Finkelhor. Like many of the treatment programmes in Canada and the USA, the core programme concentrates on encouraging offenders to take responsibility for their offences and aims to break down lies and distortions which both justify their actions to themselves and promote later offending. The initial sessions examine the stereotypes offenders have about relationships and the norms of sexual behaviour, and move on to look at the effect of offending on victims of sexual crime. This is then applied to offenders' own experiences and offences.

The second half of the programme focuses on relapse prevention. Offenders are encouraged to examine the circumstances which led up to their offending using an 'offence cycle' model.[11] The group draws up offence cycles for each of its number, identifying particularly high-risk situations (such as drinking to excess or socializing with children) which each offender needs to avoid. Each offender constructs a strategy for defusing high-risk situations. All this is documented and a copy is sent to the supervising probation officer after the prisoner's release.[12]

Unlike the core programme, the extended programme involves a high level of specialist input and individual work. It was intended for offenders 'who represented the greatest risk' and aimed to tackle offenders' needs at a far more individualized level. The precise areas of an offender's functioning to be addressed – and hence the method to be used – would vary according to the results of the assessment process. Some offenders, particularly rapists, might require work on social skills, alcohol or drug abuse, or temper control, which could be addressed by means of groups run by non-specialist staff. Others, such as habitual paedophiles, might show signs of deviant sexual arousal; these would require more specialist input by psychologists.

From the perspective of the Prison Service, this initiative was a simple method of co-ordinating and structuring the ramshackle provision that was already in place. However, in his speech to the Suzy Lamplugh Trust, Kenneth Baker was unambiguous in placing the decision to expand treatment for sex offenders in the context of public opinion:

> Sexual crime poses a difficult challenge. The courts have been taking an increasingly severe view of serious sexual crime. They have rightly made it clear that the public is entitled to expect to be protected from dangerous offenders. But most sexual offenders, however long their sentence, will eventually return to the community. They need to learn how to cope with the difficulties and temptations which they will face. The public should be able to have confidence in the arrangements for dealing with sex offenders both in custody and the community.[13]

This appeal to public opinion was backed up by a claim that the initiative would deliver significant reductions in the level of sexual crime. In the press release issued after his speech, Kenneth Baker argued that 'treatment programmes of this kind can reduce sexual recidivism by about half'.[14]

Informally, Ministers let it be known that unless significant reductions in the recidivism rate were achieved within five years, the initiative would be ended.[15]

FROM THEORY TO PRACTICE

Despite this public commitment to the initiative, there was a signal failure on the part of the Government to provide any increase in resources to cover the costs of the programmes. The lack of any mention of resources in the Home Secretary's speech prompted questions in both Houses of Parliament. However, the Government was adamant that no additional resources would be provided. Challenged in a House of Lords debate in November 1991, Viscount Astor was explicit: resources to run the treatment programme would have to be found from within existing resources by means of 'efficiency savings' and the general year-on-year Prison Service allocation in the PES round.[16]

To a large degree, the assumption that there would be no increase in resources had coloured the design of the initiative: the decision to centre the core programme around groups run by existing non-specialist prison staff was explicitly designed to limit the need for expensive specialist input.[17] However, the success of the initiative demanded that resources be increased to cover the recruitment and retention of the significant number of specialist staff needed to supervise the programmes and to carry out certain aspects of the programmes – such as the measurement of sexual arousal – which were unsuitable for non-specialists.

Moreover, although the initiative was intended to depend primarily on existing staff, those staff had to be freed from their normal duties both for initial training and in order to deliver the programmes themselves. However, the introduction of the initiative came at a time when the prison system was already overstretched by persistent overcrowding, by the cuts in prison officer hours consequent on the Fresh Start staffing agreement, and by the comprehensive programme of reforms ushered in by the Woolf Report and the 1991 Government White Paper *Custody Care and Justice*. The pressures which these factors put on prison officer time rendered the delivery of basic prison regimes difficult, let alone the undertaking of complex treatment initiatives. These factors particularly weighed upon local prisons such as Wandsworth, Wormwood Scrubs and Feltham Young Offenders' Institution (YOI), which suffered the highest levels of overcrowding.

The effect of the refusal to increase resources rendered the full implementation of the original proposal impossible. Changes had to be made to the original line-up of participating institutions. Aylesbury YOI, a prison which had long operated as a specialist facility for young male sex offenders and which had been identified as the intended assessment centre for young offenders, withdrew from the programme almost immediately because it was unable to supply the staff necessary to take part. The existing sex offender treatment groups at Aylesbury were also brought to an end. Featherstone experienced similar problems and withdrew. Wandsworth, a prison housing up to 280 sex offenders in G, H and K wings, felt unable to carry out its proposed role as an assessment centre and provider of the extended programme, limiting itself to running the core programme alone for the first year. Not all the changes were withdrawals: Whitemoor, the new dispersal prison in Cambridgeshire which opened in late 1991, joined the initiative as an assessment centre.

The pressures also affected the speed with which individual prisons were able to implement the initiative. For prisons such as Grendon, Littlehey and Wormwood Scrubs, where sex offender treatment had been a reality for some time, the initiative merely gave authority to their existing practices. In others, such as Whatton, Wakefield and Dartmoor, programmes were expanded without much difficulty. However, many other prisons struggled to free up staff and facilities to meet the challenge of their new roles. Maidstone, a prison intended to function as an assessment centre, was unable to change shift patterns to allow its uniformed staff to attend the training session given by Professor Bill Marshall, the moving spirit behind the treatment programmes in Canada and New Zealand. Their full participation in the programmes was consequently delayed. Full Sutton's momentum was halted when three of the four uniformed staff who had been trained to run the programmes were transferred from the prison. In Albany, four of the seven staff trained to run the core programmes left before the pilot programme began, delaying the pilot programme and rendering progress towards the assessment and extended programmes impossible.

The result of these problems was to slow the speed of implementation. The original intention of the Home Office had been to begin the programmes in the autumn of 1991; by the end of 1992, the programmes would be operating in all twenty prisons. However, by the autumn of 1992, the number of prisons participating in the initiative had been reduced to eighteen. Although Whitemoor had been an addition to the programmes, Aylesbury, Feltham and Featherstone had vanished from the list, and the women's prison due to participate had yet to be identified. Only fourteen of the prisons had begun to pilot the core programme, which had yet even to be evaluated. The written material for the full assessment and extended programme had not yet been finalized. These programmes, requiring specialist input and one-to-one counselling, would be far more resource-intensive than the core programme.

The necessity of increasing resources became evident even to the Home Office. In a paper circulated to the governors of the participating prisons in July 1992, Eddie Guy of DIP2 admitted:

> The pilot core programmes have been introduced largely by prioritising existing resources. There is nothing wrong with that. Prison establishments holding large numbers of sex offenders should be giving a higher priority within their regimes to work to tackle offending behaviour than many other regime activities. But, as the strategy made clear, one of the principal reasons, historically, for the failure of rehabilitative treatment programmes is inadequate resources.

The full implementation of assessment and the extended programmes *and* the extension of the programmes to greater
numbers of sex offenders, we believe, would require additional resources and we have sought to quantify these in the
current PES round. Clearly this is not a matter which can be
determined at this time, and the resources allocated for this
work must be judged against other Prison Service (and
Government) priorities.[18]

However, as the same letter revealed, the lack of resources had
not simply affected the identity of the participating prisons and
the speed of implementation; it had also affected the scope of the
initiative. The Strategy Document had been clear about who was
to be offered treatment:

It will not be practicable – at least initially – to offer treatment
programmes to all sex offenders who want or need them. The
strategy is based in part upon giving priority to those serving
four years or more . . . But the strategy is not exclusive.
Amongst those prisoners serving less than four years will be
some very dangerous men, with many victims and engaged in
an escalating pattern of deviant behaviour. Those who can
readily be identified as at high risk of re-offending . . . will be
assessed for treatment, and sentence planning will be introduced for all sex offenders.[19]

However, by July 1992, it had become clear that the resources
available could not guarantee treatment for all prisoners serving
over four years. Prisons such as Albany and Wandsworth were
able to run one or two groups at a time, each dealing with six or
eight prisoners, repeating the exercise every four or six months.
However, this would scarcely meet the demand. The commitment to treating all offenders serving over four years was therefore significantly watered down:

we intend progressively to seek to assess and offer programmes to *all* convicted of the most serious offences (i.e.
serving from 7 years to life imprisonment) . . . Those serving
between 4 and 7 years will also be assessed and a significant
proportion will be given the opportunity to take part in programmes. Those serving less than 4 years will initially only be
given high priority if they are a particularly high risk.[20]

This change is all the more significant given the fact that just 35 per cent of all sentenced sex offenders are sentenced to under four years. Moving the sentence criterion to seven years has the effect of excluding some 600 additional offenders from the priority group. More than half of all imprisoned sex offenders will now be ineligible for priority treatment and will have to wait for a place to become available.

Even given the new limitations, it was likely that some prisons would struggle. According to the prison's senior psychologist, Albany could expect to receive 100 or so eligible prisoners every year for assessment. Assuming forty of those prisoners will refuse to participate in the programme, Albany would still be required to run eight core groups a year, each staffed by a minimum of two trained staff. To do even that, without running any extended treatment programmes, he estimated that two additional psychologists and six additional, properly trained staff would be needed. Many offenders will have to wait some considerable time before they are offered treatment.[21]

In the short term, the inability of the prisons to provide treatment for all the offenders presented to them immediately means that some prisoners with only a short time to serve will not receive treatment. The Prison Service DIP2 instructions are that:

Within this group [i.e. seven years and over], cases will be prioritised, having regard to the length of time left to serve (i.e. is there sufficient time to deliver a meaningful programme) and closeness to release (i.e. we give highest priority to those who are nearest their expected release date).[22]

TIMING AND EVALUATION

The policy of giving priority to prisoners nearing the end of their sentence is only temporary. The intention, expressed in the Strategy Document and reiterated in the DIP2 letter, is that offenders are to be offered treatment as soon as possible after sentence rather than at the end. Two arguments are used to justify this approach. First, the longer sex offenders are in prison without treatment, the more likely they are to build up strong defence mechanisms which may render treatment more difficult. The persecution which they suffer at the hands of other prisoners, and the influence of their peers, may exacerbate their tendency to minimize and distort their offences. Second, and on a more practical level, the resources to run the extended programmes are only to be found in dispersal and long-term prisons, which usually hold offenders at the start rather than at the end of their sentences.[23]

This approach has been strongly criticized. Professor Bill Marshall was invited to England at a late stage in the planning of the British initiative to train the staff who were to participate. Although Professor Marshall had few criticisms of the content of the programmes, he sought a meeting in November 1991 with the Director of Inmate Programmes, Brian Emes, to protest about the timing of the treatment. Professor Marshall argued that it was futile to expect the effects of treatment to be sufficiently resilient to last from the beginning of a prisoner's sentence until that offender was finally released. An offender returned from treatment into the normal atmosphere of a prison landing or VPU would begin to lose empathy for the victim and absorb once again the beliefs which the programmes were designed to counter. Moreover, a relapse prevention strategy designed at the start of offenders' sentences might be irrelevant to their needs by the time they were released.

These arguments were not enough to persuade the Prison Service to change the policy. However, it is now intended to create a 'booster' programme to be run at Leyhill open prison for previously treated sex offenders nearing release. Nevertheless, a programme run in a single prison will be unable to offer a refresher course to more than a few offenders.

The other major feature of the initiative's design that raised concern was the plans for evaluation. Despite their public show of confidence about the effectiveness of the programmes, Ministers were anxious that the effectiveness could be demonstrated. Officials therefore decided on a policy of random allocation of some offenders to core or extended programmes and some to 'no treatment' in order to provide control groups for evaluation purposes. However, as Professor Marshall argued in a letter to Brian Emes in December 1991, this policy would have serious implications.

> The worst component of this design, however, and the one that is ethically most reprehensible never mind its political bombshell character, concerns the deliberate allocation of dangerous

offenders to either no treatment at all or to treatment that has been determined to be less than they need. Not only does this truly bizarre design have very serious ethical problems (in particular those who suffer, or may potentially suffer, at the hands of those offenders, do not have any say in the decision process – no ethics committee I can conceive of would ever approve such a programme) and a host of scary political implications, it also has disastrous implications for staff morale and operating practices.[24]

Despite Professor Marshall's pressure, there appears to have been little recognition on the part of the Prison Service of the ethical difficulties of what was being planned. What seems to have hit home was the political consequences of the policy of random allocation:

> This [policy] has been criticised on the grounds of the consequences for the offender, but also for potential future victims. While some of the criticisms have been overstated, we accept that evaluation arrangements which make no concessions to such sensibilities would be very difficult to sustain publicly.[25]

Fortunately, the inability of the Prison Service to offer treatment to all those assessed as needing it rendered arguments about random allocation somewhat academic. In practice, those offenders who had too little time left in prison for treatment to take place, or who had been unable to obtain a place on a programme, provided a more than adequate control group.

RECRUITING SUPPORT

Further worries centred on the potential effect of the prison culture on the programmes themselves. The all-pervasive macho atmosphere in many prisons appears to reinforce rather than undermine the myths which sustain sexual crime. Particular concern was expressed by the Prison Reform Trust in its review of the progress of the initiative *Beyond Containment* about the identity of some of the assessment prisons. Wandsworth, Dartmoor and Albany, the Trust argued, were prisons with reputations as punishment prisons, where relationships between staff and prisoners were traditionally marked by suspicion and hatred. The atmosphere in those prisons would not foster the mutual understanding and support that would be necessary for the success of the programmes.

However, to a large degree those fears proved groundless. While there was some evidence of prison officers exhibiting punitive and unhelpful attitudes, these were usually staff working not in the VPUs or Rule 43 units but elsewhere in the prison. At Dartmoor, the sex offender treatment programmes, far from being undermined by the punitive attitudes of many staff, acted as a spur to officers in the rest of the prison to set up groups to tackle issues such as temper control. At Wandsworth, an initiative designed to explain the rationale behind the programmes ensured the support of staff not involved in them. Only at Albany was there any significant sign of the programmes being undermined by staff.

However, the attitude of some prisoners was less welcoming. The programmes demanded that the participation of prisoners was voluntary; the groupwork model being employed rendered the participation of unmotivated offenders potentially destructive. The Woolf Inquiry concluded: 'We can confirm from the evidence they provided, that many sex offenders appear anxious to receive and co-operate with treatment.'[26] However, in practice, the reaction to the programmes varied from prison to prison. In Dartmoor, prisoners were queuing up for treatment – by September 1992, the waiting list for treatment stretched to summer 1993. However, in Wandsworth, there was a struggle even to recruit a sufficient number of prisoners to run the pilot core programmes.

To some degree, this reluctance on the part of prisoners to come forward for treatment was understandable, reflecting a traditional prisoner cynicism and lack of trust in staff initiatives. In many prisoners too, there was a refusal to accept that they had any need of treatment, either because they denied their guilt, or because they believed that they did not need any help in stopping offending. However, in some cases, it reflected an ideological belief that there was nothing wrong with sexual crime. The committed paedophiles in long-term Rule 43 units or VPUs who espouse this belief often create powerful subcultures resistent to any attempts to challenge offending. When the treatment programmes were first introduced in Whitemoor in January 1992, there were even gang-fights between sex offenders wanting to participate and others who regarded them as apostates. Pressures could also be applied in more subtle ways. Some prisoners participating in the programmes privately reported that efforts were made by other prisoners to ridicule and undermine the message of the treatment groups. In one case, a prisoner in a treatment group was being sexually assaulted by his cell-mate. These pressures inevitably would have an impact on prisoners' motivation to participate.[27]

Against these disincentives to participate was set the powerful incentive of parole. No formal, explicit connection with the parole system was made in any of the literature relating to the initiative. However, it can hardly have been coincidence that the original cut-off point for participation in the programmes was set at four years, the point at which the 1991 Criminal Justice Act laid down that parole became discretionary rather than automatic. There is little doubt that there was a deliberate, if unspoken, decision to use the possibility of a favourable parole decision as an incentive for prisoners to participate in the programmes. Certainly that was the perception of many prisoners.

However, while parole may have been an incentive to participate in the programmes, in many cases it acted as a disincentive to participate fully. The programmes seek to encourage offenders to examine their behaviour openly and honestly, and to develop strategies to minimize the possibility of reoffending. However, the indications are that many offenders have committed more offences than those of which they have been convicted. For them, being honest and open about their past behaviour would at best risk identifying themselves as more dangerous than had appeared from their official record, and at worst would lay them open to criminal prosecution. In any event, their chances of parole would be better served by hiding their offences while seeking to convince those running the programmes of their willingness to change.

This problem poses a real dilemma for those running the initiative. At best, they can hope to persuade prisoners that their long-term interests lie in full participation. They will also have to be skilled at identifying those prisoners who are continuing to conceal the truth. However, since the lure of parole will continue to be vital to prisoners' motivation, the policy of the Parole Board towards the prisoners who have participated in the programmes is crucial. Parole Board policy is to use the criterion of 'dangerousness' to determine whether or not a prisoner should be released. This could well operate against a prisoner who has disclosed previously unknown offences during treatment. On the other hand, the Parole Board may judge that a prisoner who has been honest in treatment is less likely to reoffend. Unless honest and open participation in the programmes is rewarded with parole, it is doubtful whether prisoners will risk being open about their offences or even participate in the programmes in any great numbers.

OUTSIDE THE PRISON GATES

The difficulties in integrating the prison programmes with the operation of the parole system is part of a wider and fundamental weakness of the sex offender treatment initiative. The initiative was, from the start, a Prison Service initiative. It was only in the summer of 1992, some eighteen months after the initiative was first planned, that a cross-departmental group was established in the Home Office to co-ordinate policy across the criminal justice system. It was only at that point that questions about sentencing, parole and the after-care of released prisoners began to be addressed. Even then, the cross-departmental group met only rarely and with little obvious effect.

These areas are fundamental to the success or failure of the treatment initiative. The interrelationship of the parole system and the initiative has been discussed. The policy of judges towards it is of equal importance. There was always a danger that the very existence of the programmes in prison might incline a sentencer to impose a custodial sentence 'so that an offender might receive treatment'. This danger is magnified by the policy of setting explicit criteria for participation based on offenders' sentence lengths. The knowledge that sex offenders could not be guaranteed treatment unless they were sentenced to four (now seven) years in prison may well incline a judge to sentence a prisoner to a longer term than might otherwise have been passed. Unless there is a genuine attempt to provide guidance for the judiciary, the treatment initiative might well increase the number and length of custodial sentences handed out to sex offenders.

Equally important is the question of the after-care provided to sex offenders who have participated in the programmes. As Chapter 4 has shown, the response of the probation service to sexual crime has in, some respects, been even more patchy and unco-ordinated than that of the prison system. However, it is important to note here that almost no attempt was made by the Prison Service and the probation service to co-ordinate their policies for the release and after-care of graduates from the treatment programmes. The long history of active participation of prison probation officers in sex offender treatment has obscured the absence of joint planning for prisoners' release. Since almost all of the participants in the programmes will be released on after-care licence, that failure is particularly striking.

The consequences of this failure of co-ordination are likely to be immense. In their initial announcement of the programmes, Ministers set great store by their likely impact upon recidivism rates. In the absence of any coherent attempt to plan for offenders' release, it is difficult to believe – no matter how successful the programmes in changing offenders' attitudes – that success can be translated properly into a significant reduction in reoffending. The prison treatment programmes attempt to change attitudes towards women and children in an environment from which women and children are largely absent. Resolutions made by offenders in prison may not easily survive the transition into the world outside without considerable support.

Any failure on the part of the initiative to live up to the expectations of Ministers would have consequences for the prison system that go far beyond sex offender treatment. For the prison system the sex offender initiative is a possible harbinger of other attempts at the rehabilitation of the offenders it is required to house. At Dartmoor, the programmes for sex offenders have inspired attempts to run programmes for drug problems, anger control, social skills and other behaviour. Similar initiatives are beginning elsewhere, and any failure of the sex offender programme would inevitably lead to their abandonment.

Chapter 7

Conclusion: doubts and difficulties

The panic about sexual crime has followed the classic pattern for such panics: the denial of the existence and extent of the problem; a growing fear as the facts become clearer; the knee-jerk response of tougher policing and harsher sentencing; and finally some small signs of a more considered and planned criminal justice response. However, it is difficult to argue that there now exists a coherent and effective policy towards sex offenders.

The panic has exposed fault-lines in our criminal justice system. The absence of a coherent policy towards sex offenders has emphasized the need for a mechanism for co-ordinating the policy of the criminal justice system. Although the police, the probation service and the prisons are all under the direct management of the Home Office, in practice they function as entirely independent bodies, implementing their own policies. The courts do not come under the jurisdiction of the Home Office at all, but are the responsibility of the Lord Chancellor's Department. Unlike many other countries, England and Wales do not have a Ministry of Justice with responsibility for co-ordinating criminal justice policy.

The weakness of this system was recognized by Lord Justice Woolf in his report on the prison riots of 1990. Woolf recommended the establishment of a Criminal Justice Consultative Committee, with representatives from all branches of the criminal justice system working together to co-ordinate policy.[1] The Consultative Committee was finally established in 1991, but by autumn 1992, the system of local committees envisaged by Woolf was not yet operating. Indeed, the thrust of Government policy is to weaken the links between the various agencies still further: the creation of a Prison Service Agency in April 1993 and the moves towards contracting out of many criminal justice functions will render co-ordination of policy ever more difficult.

The panic has also exposed the culture within the criminal justice agencies of weak central management and autonomous practitioners. Policing policy is made not by Ministers or the Home Office, but by the individual Chief Constables. The probation service consists of fifty-five independent services, each with its own set of priorities. The Prison Service is moving increasingly towards a model which will see policy in each prison being decided by the prison governor. Also magistrates and judges view any attempt to regulate or monitor their decision-making as an attack on judicial independence.

The furore over sexual crime has therefore made demands upon the criminal justice system which the system has been unable to meet. The unmanaged nature of the system has left its practice to be driven by the enthusiasms or prejudices of individuals. Practice has varied wildly from agency to agency, from individual to individual. Some have embraced the opportunity to create innovative and positive schemes for dealing with offenders. Others have colluded with offenders or connived at brutal and punitive responses to them.

Despite these variations, the overall effect of the panic is clear. Sexual crime is now treated more seriously by criminal justice practitioners, and sex offenders are increasingly at risk of harsh penal sanctions. Just as significantly, the campaigners for treatment for sex offenders have succeeded in ensuring that the delivery of programmes for sex offenders is at the centre of both the probation and the prison response to sexual crime.

But this is not necessarily a matter for unalloyed rejoicing. The panic has exposed the limited nature of our knowledge of the causes of sexual offending or the characteristics of most offenders. It is axiomatic that we know next to nothing about the causes of all crimes and the motivation of any offender. However, the paucity of good-quality research on sexual crime and well-tested treatment methods for sexual offenders has made the development of policy difficult even for the motivated and able criminal justice practitioners.

In this, practitioners have not been helped by the eagerness of some researchers to make questionable or simplistic claims about their findings. It is difficult to read the research without being made aware of the fragility of many of the accepted canons of faith regarding sexual crime. The beliefs that all rapists are motivated primarily by anger and hatred of women, that survivors of sexual crime always experience long-lasting psychological damage, that sexual crime is only committed by men, and that the victims are only women and children, can rely on little in the way of support from the research. Even the accepted belief that all sex offenders are unusually prone to denial and distortion can be questioned: most people would lie and minimize their guilt if questioned by someone in authority about things of which they were very ashamed – particularly if those things are related to sex.

EFFECTIVENESS OF TREATMENT

This ignorance raises important questions about the priority given by the probation service and the prison system to delivering sex offender treatment programmes. The effectiveness of any treatment methods in actually reducing the likelihood of sex offenders committing future crimes is a matter for some debate. In many cases, no outcome studies have been done to assess the effectiveness of the treatments; this is particularly true of probation and prison-based treatment programmes.[2] In many cases, too, the research that has been carried out is inadequate or seriously flawed. Studies have been badly designed; insufficient samples have been studied and insufficient follow-up times employed; results have not been properly analysed and the basis on which conclusions have been reached is often obscure. Even when such research methods are properly employed, it is rarely easy to compare one study with another.[3]

Indeed, it is doubtful whether it is even possible to devise any study which could produce accurate outcome measures for the effectiveness of treatment methods. Any attempt to measure how far treatments are successful in preventing reoffending is fraught with difficulties. Any study which takes as its measure of success whether or not offenders who have passed through the treatment programme have been reconvicted of a further sex offence is rendered almost meaningless by the fact that, as Chapter 2 showed, only a very small proportion of sexual offences are ever reported to the police, and even fewer result in a successful prosecution. The fact that 'treated' offenders have not been reconvicted is no guarantee that they have not reoffended.

Faced by those difficulties, some studies rely instead on self-reporting of offending by the offenders. However, given the apparent tendency of many sex offenders to deny or minimize their offending, and the understandable disinclination of anyone to admit to criminal behaviour, the results of self-report studies cannot be trusted.

Some researchers therefore eschew reoffending as a measure of success, and attempt instead to measure how far their programmes are successful in altering offenders' patterns of arousal. Particular claims have been made about the use of the penile plethysmograph. This is a small, mercury-filled loop which is placed over the subject's penis; the offender is then subjected to specific sexual stimuli (such as being shown pictures of children or being played audio-tapes of a rape apparently taking place) and the plethysmograph measures the engorgement of the penis with blood (and hence arousal).

However, this technique is not without both practical and theoretical problems. First, it is invasive and difficult to use: offenders have reported that the process of putting on the plethysmograph is extremely embarrassing. Second, its results are not always accurate: its use as the basis of sex offender treatment programmes in Wormwood Scrubs prison in the early 1980s was discontinued after it was discovered that prisoners were masturbating shortly before being tested in order to depress the readings.

The third problem is the most serious. Even if the plethysmograph does provide an accurate measure of an offender's arousal, that is far from providing us with a measure of whether or not the offenders will reoffend. What matters is not whether or not offenders are aroused by images of children or scenes of rape. What matters is whether offenders abuse children or commit rape. Some offenders may continue to be aroused despite the treatment they achieve, but will no longer abuse. Others may show a reduced pattern of arousal after treatment, but may continue to abuse. Measuring arousal may provide useful information, but such measures should not be the sole criterion by which the success of sex offender treatments is assessed.

For these reasons, the natural tendency of those engaging in particular methods of treatment for sex offenders to claim that their treatment is successful should be met with considerable suspicion. Indeed, in an analysis of the outcomes of forty-two studies which met their stringent criteria for inclusion (many others were judged flawed or incomplete, and discarded), Furby *et al.* concluded that:

> We can at least say with confidence that there is no evidence that treatment effectively reduces sex offender recidivism.[4]

Such a statement must not, of course, be taken to mean that no treatment can be effective in reducing recidivism, or even that none of the treatments considered actually was effective. Some sex offender treatments may actually reduce recidivism; it is just that, on Furby's analysis, they have failed to prove their effectiveness.

However, Furby's somewhat depressing conclusion has not gone unchallenged. Critics have pointed out that Furby's survey was published in January 1989 and only covered studies undertaken before that date. Since one of their criteria for inclusion was that sufficient follow-up time had elapsed since treatment, the treatment methods they examined do not necessarily represent the most up-to-date concepts on the most effective treatment (not that we can expect treatments to be better just because they are more up-to-date). The last ten years has shown a doubling of research into sexual offending, and it is entirely possible that the more modern treatment methods *are* more effective.

The most striking challenge to Furby's conclusions has come from Bill Marshall. In a paper written with colleagues from New Zealand and Canada,[5] Marshall reviewed the recidivism rates for various types of treatments. Physical interventions (psycho-surgery, castration and pharmacology) proved of limited effectiveness, with the exception of treatments which combined the prescribing of anti-androgen drugs to reduce arousal with programmes focusing on offenders' behaviour. Of the psychological treatments, by far the best results came from programmes from the cognitive/behavioural school, some of which reduced recidivism rates by up to half. Marshall and colleagues' conclusions were up-beat:

> In our review of the literature, we have attempted to answer the question: 'Can sex offenders be effectively treated so as to reduce subsequent recidivism?' We believe that the evidence provides an unequivocally positive answer to this question.

Nevertheless, Marshall added one caveat. Not all treatment programmes – indeed, not all programmes from the cognitive/behavioural school – are effective with all offenders and in all settings. In particular, while the programmes appear relatively successful with exhibitionists and child molesters, the recidivism rates for rapists remain stubbornly high. Nor can any programme be 100 per cent successful with all offenders: some failures are inevitable.

The debate between Marshall's positivism and Furby's scepticism shows that to advocate treatment for sex offenders is as yet a doctrine of hope, rather than of experience. There are some indications that it is possible to reform sex offenders, to put them through programmes which will guarantee that fewer of them will reoffend after they have been treated than would have been the case had they not been treated. However, there is still room for doubt. None of this means that the focus of penal policy has been wrong. However, there are clear dangers in basing policy on programmes which have not yet proved themselves. Today's accepted wisdom is tomorrow's half-baked theory.

MONSTERS AND BEASTS

What is needed is a cool examination of the nature of sexual crime and the criminal justice response to it. However, the nature of the panic about sexual crime has discouraged such an analysis of the phenomenon of sexual offending. A crude stereotype of a violent, calculating and perpetually dangerous sexual offender has been built up in the popular press and, to a worrying level, in 'respectable' writing about sexual crime. This stereotype may be true for an important minority of sexual offenders, but its existence militates against any attempt to assess how far individual offenders pose a continuing danger to society and how far there is scope for diverting offenders from the criminal justice system altogether. Similarly, this image of sex offender as monster hides the reality: sexual crime is committed by 'normal' people in 'normal' homes, as well as by disturbed and violent men in dark alleyways.

The image of sex offender as beast or monster sanctions punitive and brutal attitudes towards sex offenders. The vehemence of the hatred for sex offenders is unmatched by attitudes to any other offenders. It can be argued that punitive attitudes also affect sex offender treatment: some sex offenders have seen the authorities' insistence on offenders taking responsibility for their offences as an attempt by a punitive criminal justice system to instil guilt in them.

The popular stereotype of sexual crime is also built upon dishonesty. It is dishonest to pretend that some women do not fantasize about rape or that some children have not seen sex with an adult as a positive experience. It is also dishonest to say that those claiming to be victims of sexual crime are always telling the truth. To admit those things is not to downplay the horrific nature of sexual crime, to excuse any individual offender, or to give licence to rapists to rape or child abusers to abuse. The creation of coherent policy demands that it be rooted in truth.

Despite those problems, the advances of the past few years have been real and positive. The changes to police and court practices, the greater understanding of the suffering of victims reflected in the sentence lengths for sexual crime, and the improved policies in the probation service and the prison system have all been welcome changes. Moreover, in some of these agencies, the necessity of planning a response to the increased number of sexual offenders coming before them has stimulated wider change: the co-operation between the Welsh probation areas in providing a sex offender hostel and the impact that the sex offender treatment programme has had on work with prisoners in Dartmoor are just two examples.

However, there are still areas of concern. All the criminal justice agencies are undergoing periods of rapid change. All are suffering the consequences of reduced levels of resourcing and increased levels of work. In most cases, the policies towards sex offenders exist only on paper, and the structural pressures on the system may preclude the paper policies becoming practice.

If that is to be avoided, those agencies will have to continue to give priority to developing their responses towards sex offenders. Yet, by nature, panics such as this are short-lived. Already there are signs that interest in sexual crime is beginning to wane and that this is affecting the development of practice. The prison sex offender treatment programme no longer enjoys the same level of Ministerial support it did in 1991. The expansion in the number of programmes in the probation service is beginning to slow. Without a continued interest in sexual crime, it is possible that practice in ten years' time may look little different from how it did ten years ago.

Notes

INTRODUCTION

1 In a 1989 survey by MORI, rape was defined as 'very serious' by 97 per cent of the population, more than either armed robbery (93 per cent) or even murder (91 per cent) (*Reader's Digest*, vol. 132, April 1989).
2 K. Smith, *Inside Time* (London: Harrap, 1989).
3 J. Rossieau, *Medieval Prostitution* (Oxford, 1988).
4 F. McLynn, *Charles Edward Stuart* (London: Routledge, 1988).
5 J. Richards, *Sex, Dissidence and Damnation* (London: Routledge, 1990).
6 T. Boyle, *Black Swine in the Sewers of Hampstead* (New York: Viking, 1989).
7 Women's Research Centre, *Recollecting Our Lives: Women's Experience of Childhood Sexual Abuse* (Vancouver: Press Gang, 1989).
8 Liz Kelly, *Surviving Sexual Violence* (Cambridge: Polity Press, 1988).
9 E. Ward, *Father Daughter Rape* (London: Women's Press, 1984).
10 M. Hough and P. Mayhew, *British Crime Surveys 1982 and 1984* (London: HMSO, 1983 and 1985).

1 BACKGROUND TO THE PHENOMENON: DEFINITIONS AND EXPLANATIONS

1 *The Independent* (20 December 1990); *Guardian* (6 March 1992).
2 However, according to Fenton Bresler in *Sex and the Law* (London: Century Hutchinson, 1988), there has been no prosecution for consensual buggery between man and wife since 1838.
3 Howard League, *Unlawful Sex* (London: Waterlow, 1985).
4 A. Dworkin, *Right-Wing Women* (London, 1983). As Roy Porter has pointed out, this is a nice feminist counterpoint to the male myth that 'all women want it really' (in S. Tomaselli and R. Porter, *Rape* (Blackwell: Oxford, 1986)).
5 J. Caputi, *The Age of Sex Crime* (London: Women's Press, 1988).
6 *The Independent* (10 January 1991).
7 *The Independent on Sunday* (29 September 1991).
8 As is the case in many European countries, in Spain sex with a

12-year-old is only legal if no trickery is used and there is no abuse of power. There is a higher age of consent – 18 – to cover such cases.

9   *Understanding Paedophilia* (London: PIE, 1977).
10 See, for example, D. Finkelhor, *Child Sexual Abuse* (New York: Free Press, 1984).
11 R. Tannahill, *Sex in History* (London: Cardinal, 1989).
12 T. Sandford, *The Sexual Aspect of Paedophile Relations* (Amsterdam: Pan/Spartacus, 1982).
13 J. Nelson, 'The impact of incest' in L. Constantine and F. Martinson (eds), *Children and Sex* (Boston: Little, Brown, 1982).
14 Finkelhor, *op. cit.*
15 See, for example, J. Herman, *Father–Daughter Incest* (Cambridge: Harvard, 1981).
16 D. Finkelhor, *op. cit.*
17 D. Finkelhor, *op. cit.*
18 D. Grubin and J. Gunn, *The Imprisoned Rapist and Rape* (London: Home Office, 1990).
19 R. Langevin, 'Defensiveness in Sex Offenders' in R. Rogers (ed.), *Clinical Assessment of Malingering and Deception* (New York: Guildford Press, 1988). Also H. Kennedy and D. Grubin, *Patterns of Denial in Sex Offenders* (submitted for publication).
20 Quoted by David Saunders-Wilson in *Beyond Containment* (London: Prison Reform Trust, 1992).
21 S. Brownmiller, *Against Our Will: Men, Women and Rape* (New York: Penguin, 1976).
22 Brownmiller, *op. cit.*
23 A. Groth and A. Burgess, 'Rape: a pseudosexual act', *International Journal for Women's Studies* 1: 207–10 (1978).
24 *The Independent* (14 December 1991).
25 The self-help organization London Survivors deals with over 1,000 referrals a year from the South East alone.
26 See R. McMullin, *Male Rape* (London: Gay Men's Press, 1990).
27 *Guardian* (5 March 1992).
28 J. Check and N. Malamuth, 'Sex role stereotyping and reactions to depictions of stranger versus acquaintance rape', *Journal of Personality and Social Psychology* 45 (1983).
29 N. Malamuth, 'Rape proclivity among males', *Journal of Social Issues* 37 (1981).
30 J. Check and N. Malamuth, 'An empirical assessment of some feminist hypotheses about rape', *International Journal of Women's Studies* 8 (1985); K. Rapaport and B. Burkhart, 'Personality and attitudinal characteristics of sexually coercive college males', *Journal of Abnormal Psychology* 93 (1984).
31 See, for example, Peggy Reeves Sanday's work on Western Sumatra in S. Tomaselli and R. Porter (eds), *Rape* (Oxford: Blackwell, 1986).
32 B. Yegedis, 'Date rape and other forced sexual encounters among college students', *Journal of Sex Education and Therapy* 12 (1986).
33 E. Kanin, 'Date rapists', *Archives of Sex Behaviour* 14 (1985).
34 There are many examples of Victorian women sexually abusing their

servant girls. One, given in Thomas Boyle's *Black Swine in the Sewers of Hampstead* (New York: Viking, 1989), records a mistress forcing a servant to eat excrement and sexually abusing her with a poker.

35 R. Thornhill and N. Thornhill, 'Human rape: an evolutionary analysis' in *Ethology and Sociobiology* (4) (1983). See also R. Thornhill, N. Thornhill and G. Dizinno in S. Tomaselli and R. Porter, *op. cit.*

36 Thornhill and Thornhill, *op. cit.*

37 Equally, this finding can reflect institutional bias in the criminal justice system. It could be argued that it is mainly poor, ill-educated and lower-class rapists who are ever caught and successfully prosecuted.

38 D. Russell, *Sexual Exploitation* (Beverly Hills, CA: Sage, 1984).

39 Groth and Burgess (1980) quoted in McMullen, *op. cit.*

40 These acts occurred in 35 per cent and 17 per cent respectively of the cases studied by Grubin and Gunn, *op. cit.*

41 In 12 per cent of the cases studied by Grubin and Gunn, *op. cit.*, for example.

42 Thornhill and Thornhill, *op. cit.*

43 R. Prentky, *Sexual Violence* (1990; unpublished, but cited in Grubin and Gunn, *op. cit.*). None of the rapists studied by Grubin and Gunn showed evidence of psychopathy.

44 K. Moyer, *The Psychobiology of Aggression* (New York: Harper & Row, 1976).

45 R. Langevin, *Erotic Preference, Gender Identity and Aggression in Men* (Hillsdale, NJ: Lawrence Erlbaum, 1984).

46 Hence Brownmiller's diatribe against Freud and his followers: 'We may thank the legacy of Freudian psychology for fostering a totally inaccurate popular conception of rape' (S. Brownmiller, *op. cit.*). For a counter-argument, see J. Forrester, 'Rape, seduction and psycho-analysis' in S. Tomaselli and R. Porter (eds), *Rape* (London: Blackwell, 1986).

47 Quoted in R. Wyre and A. Swift, *Women, Men and Rape* (London: Hodder & Stoughton, 1990).

48 J. Coid 'Alcohol, rape and sexual assault' in P. Brain (ed.), *Alcohol and Aggression* (London: Croom Helm, 1986).

49 R. Langevin, *Sexual Strands* (Hillsdale, NJ: Lawrence Erlbaum, 1983).

50 P. Bart and P. O'Brien, *Stopping Rape: Successful Survival Strategies*, The Athene Series (Oxford: Pergamon Press, 1985).

51 Howells (1981).

52 A. Burgess (ed.), *Child Pornography and Sex Rings* (Lexington, MA: Lexington Books, 1984).

53 Groth and Burgess (1979).

54 I. Cooper and B. Cormier, 'Inter-generational transmission of incest', *Canadian Journal of Psychiatry* 27 (1982).

55 Grubin and Gunn, *op. cit.*

56 W. Marshall and H. Barbaree, 'An integrated theory of the etiology of sexual offending' in W. Marshall, D. Laws and H. Barbaree, *Handbook of Sexual Assault* (London: Plenum Press, 1990).

57 D. Finkelhor, *op. cit.*

58 C. Glasman, *New Law Journal* (14 July 1989).
59 See D. Scully and J. Marolla, 'Convicted rapists' vocabulary of motive: excuses and justifications' in *Social Problems* 31 (1984).
60 *The Independent* (7 December 1992). The young man, a shy student with few social skills, had taken to masturbating in or near the car, being particularly obsessed with the exhaust.
61 D. Perkins, 'Social skills training with dangerous offenders' in *Making Social Skills Effective: Papers on First Annual SST Conference* (Leicester: Association for Psychological Therapies, 1987).
62 L. Warwick, *Community based work with sex offenders: the probation service response*, UEA Social Work Monograph (1991).
63 See, for example, C. White, 'TA with sex offenders', *Probation Journal* (March 1992).
64 *Guardian* (4 December 1990).
65 *Cutting Edge*, broadcast on 7 December 1992.
66 A. Cooper, 'Progestogen in the treatment of male sex offenders: a review', *Canadian Journal of Psychiatry* 31 (1986).
67 For a forceful rejection of chemical castration, see the review of European research studies by N. Heim and C. Hursch, 'Castration for sex offenders: treatment or punishment?', *Archives of Sexual Behaviour* 8 (1979).

2 FROM CRIME TO CONVICTION

1 C. Nash and D. West, 'The sexual molestation of young girls' in D. West (ed.), *Sexual Victimisation* (London: Gower Press, 1985).
2 BBC Childwatch Survey (1986).
3 Women Against Rape, *Ask Any Woman* (London: Women Against Rape, 1982).
4 *Company* magazine survey (September 1989).
5 Home Office Standing Committee on Crime Prevention, *Fear of Crime* (London: Home Office, 1990).
6 R. McMullen, *Male Rape* (London: Gay Men's Press, 1990).
7 R. Wyre and A. Swift, *Men, Women and Rape* (London: Hodder & Stoughton, 1990).
8 J. La Fontaine, *Child Sexual Abuse: An ESRC Research Briefing* (ESRC, 1988).
9 R.E. Hall, *Ask Any Woman: A London inquiry into rape and sexual assault* (Bristol: Women Against Rape, 1985). The methodology used in this survey has been criticized by McLean, *British Journal of Criminology* 25: 390 (1985).
10 Hall, *op. cit.*
11 *Ibid.*
12 A. Snare, 'Sexual Violence against Women' in *Sexual Behaviour and Attitudes and their Implication for Criminal Law*, Report of 15th Criminological Research Conference Strasbourg (Council of Europe, 1983).
13 WAR, *op. cit.* The WAR study found that 79 per cent of women trying to leave rapist husbands were trapped in that situation by lack of money or housing.

14 P.R. Wilson, *The Other Side of Rape* (Queensland, 1978).
15 *The Times* (12 August 1991).
16 K. Painter, 'Wife rape, sex, law and marriage' in *Criminal Justice Matters No. 5* (London: ISTD, 1991).
17 *The Times* (24 October 1991).
18 *The Times* (25 October 1991).
19 *The Independent* (25 October 1991).
20 WAR, *op. cit.*
21 See for example *Report of the Advisory Group on the Law of Rape*, Cmnd 6352 (London: Home Office, 1975).
22 The London Rape Crisis Centre report *Strength in Numbers* (London, 1987) found that two-thirds of those who reported rapes to the police characterized the police attitude as unsympathetic.
23 *Guardian* (25 January 1985).
24 Written answer to Parliamentary Question, *Hansard c. 257*, (25 October 1990).
25 In a survey reported in *Police Review*, 31 May 1991. Zuzanna Adler found that of a sample of 103 women who reported rape or serious sexual assault during 1990–1, no less than 79 per cent were treated better than they expected. Indeed, the attitudes exhibited by police officers seemed to be far better than those exhibited by some of the examining doctors. Of the sample, 70 per cent had been seen in victim examination suites.
26 In the London Rape Crisis Centre study, old-style committals were used in half the cases that came to trial (*op. cit.*).
27 Z. Adler, 'The Reality of Rape Trials' in *New Society* 4(ii) (1982).
28 See, for example, T. Gibbens and I. Prince, *Child Victims of Sex Offences* (London: Institute for the Study and Treatment of Delinquency, 1963).
29 Both examples quoted in F. Bresler, *Sex and the Law* (London: Hutchinson, 1988). Unfortunately, Mr Bresler does not date the first of the two.
30 *Report of the Advisory Group on the Law of Rape*, Cmnd 3252 (London: HMSO, 1976).
31 K. Soothill and S. Walby, *Sex Crime in the News* (London: Routledge, 1991).
32 M. Hough and P. Mayhew, *The British Crime Survey: First Report*, Home Office Research Study 76 (London: HMSO, 1985); P. Mayhew, D. Elliott and L. Dowds, *The 1988 British Crime Survey*, Home Office Research Study 111 (London: HMSO, 1989).
33 *The Independent* (14 February 1991).
34 See K. Soothill and S. Walby, *op cit.*
35 *Evening Standard* (13 September 1990).
36 Written answer, *Hansard c. 537* (22 October 1991).
37 *Guardian* (4 October 1991).
38 At the time of writing, Leicestershire and South Yorkshire continue to have active bars to homosexual employment in the police force.
39 *The Independent* (12 November 1991).
40 *Capital Gay* (7 December 1990.

41 *Daily Telegraph* (12 September 1991).
42 Paper presented at a conference *Investigating Child Sexual Abuse* on 10 December 1990 by Sue Conroy from Dept of Sociology, University of Surrey. However, the survey emphasized that practice was patchy across the country and beset by resource difficulties and differences in culture between the organizations.
43 *Guardian* (12 July 1991).
44 M. Hough and P. Mayhew, *op. cit.*, and P. Mayhew, D. Elliott and L. Dowds, *op. cit.*
45 D. Russell, 'The prevalence and incidence of forcible rape and attempted rape of females', *Victimology: An International Journal* 7(1–4) (1982); D. Russell and N. Howell, 'The prevalence of rape in the United States revisited', *Signs: Journal of Women in Culture and Society* 8 (1983).
46 Women Against Rape, *Ask Any Woman* (London, 1982).
47 *Company* (September 1989).
48 R. McMullen, *op. cit.*
49 *Guardian* (23 July 1991).
50 G. Wyatt, 'The sexual abuse of Afro-American and white American women in childhood', *Child Abuse and Neglect* 9 (1985).
51 G. Fritz, K. Stoll and N. Wagner, 'A comparison of males and females who were molested as children', *Journal of Sex and Marital Therapy* 7 (1984).
52 A. Baker and S. Duncan, 'Child sexual abuse: a study of prevalence in Great Britain', *Child Abuse and Neglect* 9 (1985).
53 C. Nash and D. West, 'Sexual molestation of young girls: a retrospective study' in D. West (ed.), *Sexual Victimization* (Aldershot: Gower, 1985).
54 L. Kelly, L. Regan and S. Burton, *An Exploratory Study of the Prevalence of Sexual Abuse in a Sample of 16–21 Year-Olds*, Child Abuse Studies Unit, Polytechnic of North London, 1991.
55 L. Smith, *Concerns About Rape*, Home Office Research Study No. 106 (London: HMSO, 1989).
56 London Rape Crisis Centre, *Strength in Numbers* (London, 1987).
57 D. Grubin and J. Gunn, *The Imprisoned Rapist and Rape* (London: Home Office, 1990).
58 L. Kelly, L. Regan and S. Burton, *op cit.*
59 *Guardian* (20 November 1991). These figures formed the basis for a Channel 4 programme, *Dispatches*, shown on the same date.
60 R. Wright, 'A note on the attribution of rape cases', *British Journal of Criminology* 24 (1984).
61 *Criminal Statistics England and Wales 1989* (London: HMSO, 1990).
62 Howard League Working Party, *Unlawful Sex* (London: Waterlow, 1985).
63 *Crown Prosecution Service Annual Report 1989–1990* (London: HMSO, 1990).
64 Butler-Sloss, *Report of an Enquiry into Child Abuse in Cleveland 1987* (London: HMSO, 1988).
65 According to the *Guardian* (20 October 1992), Nottingham Social

Services finally agreed to pay for the treatment of an unconvicted child abuser after a judge, Mr Justice Ward, criticized the council's initial refusal to pay as 'irresponsible'. However, Social Services pointed out that although under the Children Act 1990 the council had a duty to take action to protect children, it had no legal responsibility to offer treatment to the abuser.

66 See, for example, D. Glaser and J. Spencer 'Sentencing, children's evidence and children's trauma', *Criminal Law Review* (June 1990).
67 A. Manchester, 'Incest and the Law' in J. Eckelaar and S. Katz (eds), *Family Violence* (Toronto: Butterworths, 1978).
68 *Criminal Statistics England and Wales 1980–1990* (London: HMSO 1981 and 1991).
69 A case in point is the Epping Forest 'satanic abuse' case which was aborted in November 1991 when the testimony of one 10-year-old witness was admitted to be unreliable by the prosecution.

3 SENTENCING: JUST DESERTS AND PUBLIC PROTECTION

1 G. Pearson, *Hooligan: A History of Respectable Fears* (London: Open University Press, 1983).
2 K. Soothill and S. Walby, *Sex Crime in the News* (London: Routledge, 1991).
3 M. Hough and P. Mayhew, *The British Crime Survey*, Home Office Research Study 76 (London: HMSO, 1983); M. Hough and P. Mayhew, *Taking Account of Crime: key findings from the 1984 British Crime Survey*, Home Office Research Study 85 (London: HMSO, 1985). The findings of the 1988 BCS about the public fear of crime have not been published.
4 Home Office Standing Committee on Crime Prevention, *Fear of Crime* (London: Home Office, 1990).
5 See, for example, the suggestion in a letter to the *Guardian* (15 November 1991) from Michael Grade that crime statistics be published only twice a year in order to lessen women's fear of rape.
6 *Daily Mail* (11 January 1985).
7 *Evening Standard* (24 February 1992).
8 *The Times* (8 February 1993).
9 *Guardian* (9 February 1987).
10 *Criminal Statistics England and Wales 1989* (London: HMSO, 1990).
11 W. Marshall, A. Eccles and H. Barbaree, 'A Three-tiered approach to the rehabilitation of incarcerated sex offenders', *Behavioural Sciences and the Law* (1992).
12 F. Bresler, *Sex and the Law* (London: Frederick Muller, 1988).
13 *The Pink Paper* (6 July 1991).
14 C. Lloyd and R. Walmsley, *Changes in Rape Offences and Sentencing*, Home Office Research Study 105 (London: HMSO, 1989).
15 *Daily Telegraph* (1 August 1991).
16 *The Independent* (9 January 1992). These arguments were supported by Professor Glanville Williams in the *Guardian* on 11 January. He

argued that since 'the stranger who pounces . . . is a greater menace to society and a greater terror to women than the known attacker', men who rape women they know should receive more lenient sentences than men who rape strangers. This view attracted concerted opposition from rape survivors (*Guardian*, 15 January).

17 *The Independent* (14 December 1991).
18 *The Times* (10 December 1990).
19 *Attorney General's Reference No. 1.*
20 *Hansard* (20 February 1991), c. 391.
21 *Van Droogenbroeck v Belgium*, 4 EHRR 443 (1982).
22 *Thynne, Wilson and Gunnell v UK* (1989).
23 *Report of the Parole Board 1989* (London: HMSO, 1990).
24 *Today* (29 July 1992).

4 SEX OFFENDERS AND PROBATION: A CHALLENGE DUCKED?

1 J. Halliday in *Report of the Tripartite Seminar 1991 on the Effective Management of Sex Offenders* (Home Office, 1991).
2 Speech by Roger Ford, Chief Probation Officer Shropshire *Report of Tripartite Seminar 'The Effective Management of Sex Offenders'* (Home Office Probation Division, 1991).
3 M. Barker and R. Morgan, 'Probation practice with sex offenders surveyed; *Probation Journal* (December 1991).
4 ACOP discussion paper *Working with Sex Offenders* (February 1992).
5 R. Martinson, 'What works? Questions and answers about prison reform', *Public Interest* 35, 1974.
6 S. Brody, *The Effectiveness of Sentencing: A Review of the Literature*, Home Office Research Study 35 (London: HMSO, 1976).
7 M. Folkard, D.E. Smith and D.D. Smith, *IMPACT: vol. II, The Results of the Experiment*, Home Office Research Study 36 (London: HMSO, 1976).
8 G. Mair, *What works – Nothing or Everything? Measuring the Effectiveness of Sentences*, Home Office Research Bulletin (London: HMSO, 1992).
9 R. Ross and P. Gendreau (eds) *Effective Correctional Treatment* (Canada: Butterworth, 1980).
10 C. Yates, 'A family affair: sexual offences, sentencing and treatment', *Journal of Child Care Law* 2 (1990).
11 The areas examined were Avon, Cornwall, Oxfordshire, Staffordshire, South Yorkshire and West Glamorgan.
12 L. Warwick, *Community Based Work with Sex Offenders*: The Probation Service Response, Social Work Monograph (UEA, 1991).
13 M. Barker and R. Morgan, 'Probation practice with sex offenders surveyed', *Probation Journal* (December 1991).
14 A short survey by questionnaire carried out by the author in October 1992.
15 HM Inspectorate of Probation, *The Work of the Probation Service with*

Sex Offenders (Home Office: London, 1991); Directerate of Inmate Programmes, *Treatment Programmes for Sex Offenders in Custody: A Strategy* (Home Office: London, 1991).
16 M. Barker and R. Morgan, *op. cit.*
17 *Ibid.*
18 *Changing Men: A Practice Guide to Working with Adult Male Sex Offenders*, Nottinghamshire Probation Service (1992).
19 M. Barker and R. Morgan, *op. cit.*
20 C. Hawkes in *Beyond Containment* (London: Prison Reform Trust, 1992).
21 M. Sabor, 'The sex offender treatment programme in prisons', *Probation Journal* (March 1992).
22 T. Morrison, 'Managing sex offenders: the challenge for managers', *Probation Journal* (September 1992).
23 *Ibid.*
24 NAPO Professional Committee guideline PP66/91.
25 ACOP, *op. cit.*
26 The need to ensure that probation officers who have been abused have the option of opting out of working with sex offenders was the subject of a resolution passed at the 1989 NAPO conference. However, there has been little subsequent progress towards the development of formal mechanisms to allow this to happen in such a way as to avoid harming the officers' careers.
27 T. Morrison, *op. cit.*
28 *Partnership in Dealing with Offenders in the Community*, Home Office Discussion Paper (1990).

5 A PRISON WITHIN A PRISON

1 Quoted in *The Independent* (15 October 1988).
2 *Ibid.*
3 *Birmingham Evening Mail* (25 September 1992).
4 *Sun* (30 November 1989). He returned to the theme on 23 October 1992. Reacting to the sentencing of James Cochrane for the rape and murder of a 4-year-old boy, he wrote: Let us pray that every day of the rest of his miserable life, this disgusting and evil rodent is subjected to the vilest of sexual assaults and then beaten senseless. There are some people for whom only a baseball bat and a rusty Stanley knife will suffice.'
5 *Hansard* (20 November 1990) col. 216.
6 See, for example, K. Smith, *Inside Time* (London: Harrap, 1989).
7 *Daily Telegraph* (29 October 1992).
8 *Daily Telegraph* (10 June 1992).
9 T. Hercules, *Labelled a Black Villain* (London: Fourth Estate, 1989).
10 See, for example, P. Turnbull, K. Dolan and G. Stimson, *Prisons HIV and AIDS: Risks and Experiences in Custodial Care* (London: AVERT, 1991).
11 Smith, *op. cit.*
12 Hercules, *op. cit.*

13 *Guardian* (5 March 1992).
14 *Report of the Working Party on the Management of Vulnerable Prisoners*, Home Office Internal document (1989).
15 Woolf Report, para. 12.196.
16 This can be found as Proposal 15.44 in the Woolf Report.
17 J. Hennessey, *A Review of the Segregation of Prisoners under Rule 43* (London: HMSO, 1986).
18 *Social Work Today* (21 September 1989).
19 *The Independent* (2 September 1991).
20 *Report of the Working Party on the Management of Vulnerable Prisoners*, Home Office internal document (1989).
21 S. Tumim, *HM Chief Inspector's Report on Parkhurst* (London: HMSO, 1988).
22 See M. Cowburn in *Beyond Containment* (London: Prison Reform Trust, 1992).
23 *Hansard* (15 June 1991).
24 R. King and K. McDermott, 'The ever-deepening crisis', *British Journal of Criminology* (1989).
25 *Home Office News Release* (29 October 1986).
26 S. Tumim, *HM Chief Inspector of Prisons Report on HMP Wandsworth* (London: HMSO, 1989).
27 Home Office Working Party, *op. cit.*
28 I. Dunbar, *A Sense of Direction* (London: Home Office, 1986).
29 See, for example, the Prison Reform Trust report *Implementing Woolf* (London: Prison Reform Trust, 1992), which surveyed the extent of the reforms prison governors had been able to implement in the light of the Woolf Report without increases in resourcing. These included such changes as increases in visiting entitlement, removal of censorship of letters, changes in mealtimes, etc.
30 Thornton in B. McGurk, D. Thornton and M. Williams, *Applying Psychology to Imprisonment* (London: HMSO, 1987).
31 *Woolf Report*, para. 12.210.
32 Home Office Working Party, *op. cit.*
33 S. Tumim, *HM Chief Inspector of Prisons' Report on Stafford* (London: HMSO, 1991).
34 *Sex Offenders In Prison* (London: Prison Reform Trust, 1989). The quotation from HM Chief Inspector of Prisons comes from the *Daily Telegraph* (10 October 1988).
35 The exception to this rule is France, where there is a growing problem with attacks on sex offenders. Russia and its neighbours have experienced similar problems in the past. In Scotland, most sex offenders (of whom there are very few compared to England and Wales) are segregated in Peterhead. Ironically, the majority of the other prisoners at Peterhead have been sent there for assaults on their peers.
36 For a description of this process, see Steve Twinn's chapter in *Beyond Containment* (London: Prison Reform Trust, 1992).
37 *HMP Wandsworth: A Model Regime*, Report on a strategic planning workshop for Wandsworth management (September 1992).
38 *The Times* (24 October 1991).

6 TREATMENT IN PRISON: ORDER OUT OF CHAOS

1 *Report of the May Committee of Inquiry into the United Kingdom Prison Services*, Cmnd 76723 (London: HMSO, 1979).
2 *Woolf Report*, para. 12.216.
3 The research was on the subject of probation involvement in sex offender treatment in prisons. One chapter of Malcolm Cowburn's research was published in a revised form in the Prison Reform Trust's report *Beyond Containment* (London: Prison Reform Trust, 1992).
4 *Sex Offenders in Prison* (London: Prison Reform Trust, 1990).
5 Although treatment initiatives were undertaken and evaluated at Oxford, at Aylesbury Young Offenders' Institution and at Styal Women's Prison during 1988 and 1989, for example, these evaluations (by J. Sandham, by P. Wilson and J. Chine, and by S. Barnett, F. Corder and D. Jehu respectively) were never published.
6 See, for example, J. Gunn, G. Robertson, S. Dell and C. Way, *Psychiatric Aspects for Imprisonment* (London: Academic Press, 1978), followed up later in G. Robertson and J. Gunn, 'A ten year follow-up of men discharged from Grendon prison', *British Journal of Psychiatry* 151 (1987). For a general account of Grendon, see Tony Parker's picture of the prison in the late 1960s, *The Frying Pan* (London: Hutchinson, 1970). Unfortunately, Elaine Gender and Elaine Players' 1989 research study on Grendon has yet to be published by the Home Office.
7 For accounts of the crisis in the Annexe, see the media coverage in *The Times* and *The Independent* (13 September 1989). A contrary view was expressed by the senior hospital officer in the unit in a letter in the POA magazine *Gatelodge* in October 1989.
8 *Sex Offenders in Prison* (London: Prison Reform Trust, 1990).
9 *Woolf Report*, paras 12.214 and 12.215 (emphasis in the original). These paragraphs were distilled into a formal proposal that 'More attention should be given to the treatment of sex offenders and to providing assistance to prevent their re-offending' (proposal 124).
10 *Treatment Programmes for Sex Offenders in Custody: A Strategy*, HM Prison Service (July 1991).
11 This model, derived loosely from Finkelhor and behavioural analysts, sees offending as part of a cycle: a trigger event leads to someone with a predilection for sexual crime beginning to think or fantasize about offending. This fantasy coheres into a concrete plan, with a selected target, and the circumstances are arranged to enable it to take place. The offence itself is followed by a post-offence reaction, such as guilt or exultation, which may promote further offending. It is noticeable that while this model need not be specific only to sexual crime – it is an analysis which could usefully be applied to all types of human behaviour.
12 This part of the programme, which should be of central importance in helping to prevent reoffending, is in practice somewhat sketchy. In only a few prisons is relapse prevention given much weight, and the relapse prevention strategies are rarely produced in a written form. Some staff have expressed doubts about how effective the

programme can be unless relapse prevention is given greater priority.

13 Kenneth Baker, *Speech to the Suzy Lamplugh Trust Conference on the Sentencing of Sex Offenders* (7 June 1991).

14 *Home Office News Release* (10 June 1991).

15 Rt Hon. Angela Rumbold MP (then Minister for State at the Home Office), personal communication.

16 *Hansard* (13 November 1991), col. 646.

17 'A core programme, *which does not require significant specialist resources,* will tackle offenders' distorted beliefs . . .', G. Guy, 'Management Summary', para 1 (vi) in *Treatment Programmes for Sex Offenders in Custody: A Strategy* (added emphasis).

18 Internal Prison Service letter, 9 July 1992 (emphasis in the original).

19 *Ibid.*

20 *Ibid.* (emphasis in the original).

21 Personal communication.

22 Internal Prison Service letter, *op. cit.*

23 Wandsworth, a poorly resourced local prison holding prisoners on remand and immediately after sentence, is one obvious exception.

24 Letter to Brian Emes, Director of Inmate Programmes, 16 December 1991.

25 Internal Prison Service letter, *op. cit.*

26 *Woolf Report*, para. 12.219.

27 Personal communication.

7 CONCLUSION: DOUBTS AND DIFFICULTIES

1 Lord Justice Woolf and Judge S. Tumim, *Report of an Inquiry into the Prison Disturbances, April 1990* (London: HMSO, 1991), Recommendation 1.

2 See HM Inspectorate of Probation, *The Work of the Probation Service with Sex Offenders* (Home Office: London, 1991); Directorate of Inmate Programmes, *Treatment Programmes for Sex Offenders in Custody: A Strategy* (Home Office: London, 1991).

3 See L. Furby, M. Weinrott and L. Blackshaw, 'Sex offender recidivism: a review', in *Psychological Bulletin*, Vol. 105, No. 1, American Psychological Association (1989).

4 Furby *et al., op. cit.*

5 W. Marshall, R. Jones, A. Ward, P. Johnston and H. Barbaree, 'Treatment outcome with sex offenders', *Clinical Psychology Review* 11 (1991).

Index